High Praise for
Cooking for Life

"WHAT WE PEOPLE WITH AIDS HAVE BEEN WAITING FOR: A POCKETBOOK FOR DEVOTEES OF GOOD FOOD AND GOOD HEALTH INCORPORATING EMINENTLY PRACTICAL TIPS FOR HIV NUTRITION."

> —Kiyoshi Kuromiya, director, Critical Path Project and author of *The Act Up Standard of Care*

"Chef Rob addresses the practical aspects of food and nutrition for HIV-positive people in warm, caring, and 'get real!' fashion. He emphasizes the important points of day-to-day living and eating. He makes it all doable. A must-have book for people living with HIV."

> —Cade Fields-Gardner, M.S., R.D./ L.D., director of services, The Cutting Edge, and author of *Nutritional Management in HIV Disease*

"There are no magical or wishful solutions here, no promotion of unproven costly remedies. Instead *Cooking for Life* offers a balanced and reassuring view of what is truly known and what can reasonably be done by almost any HIV-positive person."

> —Martin Delaney, director, Project Inform

"*COOKING FOR LIFE* STANDS UP TO THE CHALLENGE OF MAINTAINING NUTRITIONAL COMPETENCE IN HIV, AND OFFERS SOLUTIONS WITH PRACTICALITY AND TENDERNESS."

> —Mary Romeyn, M.D., author of *Nutrition and HIV*

COOKING FOR LIFE

A Guide to Nutrition and Food Safety
for the HIV-Positive Community

Robert H. Lehmann

with medical advisors
Norma Muurahainen, M.D., Ph.D.
Peggi Guenter, Ph.D., R.N., C.N.S.N.
Margaret Cauterucci, R.D.

A Dell Trade Paperback

A DELL TRADE PAPERBACK

Published by
Dell Publishing
a division of
Bantam Doubleday Dell Publishing Group, Inc.
1540 Broadway
New York, New York 10036

Library of Congress Cataloging in Publication Data
Lehmann, Robert H.
    Cooking for life : a guide to nutrition and food safety for the
HIV-positive community / by Robert H. Lehmann.
        p.   cm.
    ISBN 0-440-50753-7
    1. AIDS (Disease)—Diet therapy.   2. AIDS (Disease)—
Nutritional aspects.   3. AIDS (Disease)—Prevention.   I. Title.
RC607.A26L435   1996
616.97'920654—dc20   96–12823
                                      CIP

Printed in the United States of America

Published simultaneously in Canada

January 1997

10 9 8 7 6 5 4 3 2 1

BVG

STATEMENT OF NONCOMPENSATED ENDORSEMENT

Products recommended in this book by specific brand name are done so because they are, to the best of my knowledge, either the most appropriate product for the situation discussed and/or are the most widely available products appropriate for the situation. I have received no compensation whatsoever from the companies involved.

*For Alex Nixon,
without whose loyal friendship
and steadfast support
this book could not
possibly, possibly exist.*

Contents

My heartfelt thanks to the following people:

To Marge Cauterucci, Peggi Guenter, and Norma Muurahainen, my three Muses of nutrition, Graces all, who just this once have been called upon to play the role of the Fates.

To Nancy Nixon, Harry Kaplan, and Carol Hart, who led this babe through the woods of Computerland.

To Gary Cohan, Sharon Finnegan, Jodie and Stephen Forrest, Debbie Gooch, my fabulous editor, Stephanie Gunning, my dear Cleora Hudson, Donald Kotler, Bill Krumbolt, Kiyoshi Kuromiya, Jane Lycens, Nancie McDermott, Angela Miller, Lisa Newbold, Dean Nichols, Richard Pooler, Jeanine Stewart, Mary Torrence, Craig Weirum, and Charles Rue Woods.

Medical Advisors

NORMA MUURAHAINEN, M.D., Ph.D.

Dr. Muurahainen is a physician who received her Ph.D. in human nutritional biochemistry from Columbia University. She is the director of HIV Nutrition Research at the Graduate Hospital, Philadelphia, Pennsylvania, and a clinical assistant professor at the University of Pennsylvania School of Medicine. Dr. Muurahainen sees HIV patients in private practice and nutritional consultation, publishes, and lectures internationally.

PEGGI GUENTER, Ph.D., R.N., C.N.S.N.*

Dr. Guenter is currently the coordinator, Nutrition Support Service, the Graduate Hospital, Philadelphia, Pennsylvania. She received her Ph.D. from the University of Pennsylvania in 1993 based on dissertation research entitled "The Impact of Nutritional Status and HIV Disease Progression on Survival in Patients with HIV Infection." She is also serving a five-year term as editor-in-chief of *Nutrition in Clinical Practice*, an official journal of the American Society for Parenteral and Enteral Nutrition.

*Certified Nutrition Support Nurse

MARGARET CAUTERUCCI, R.D.

Mrs. Cauterucci developed and conducted a proactive HIV/Nutrition component for the Early Intervention Program of Philadelphia's Southeast Health Center by which hundreds of HIV-positive individuals received nutritional counseling as part of their routine medical care. As the mother of three sons—two of whom have hemophilia—she has a personal commitment to the concerns and issues surrounding HIV. Mrs. Cauterucci takes much pride that her work with HIV/nutrition has always been funded by the legacy of a young man with hemophilia: Ryan White.

COOKING FOR LIFE

Foreword
by Donald P. Kotler, M.D.

As we advance into the second decade of the AIDS epidemic, much has changed. Though great strides have been made in medical treatments and therapies, this plague has outpaced them. At the same time we have seen hopes for a completely effective treatment or vaccine diminish. The controversy over antiretrovirals proceeds unabated and such treatment is not even an option for many people. After a decade of annual meetings the International Conference on AIDS, by far the largest of its kind, has elected to meet only biennially. What can be done?

The Hippocratic oath admonishes: "First, do no harm." We must take the tools we *do* have, which *do* work, and use them. Malnutrition is a crippling problem in the AIDS community. Nutrition and food safety are not cures for HIV, but they are among the most effective and least utilized weapons in our fight against it. Conscientiousness about nutrition is growing in both the public and professional sectors, due in large part to its emerging role as a clear winner in the AIDS crisis; it is a response that has no toxicity, that embraces the concerns of empowerment and quality of life, and without which optimal health is impossible.

Too often, in light of the lack of research-informed and detailed nutritional guidance, people living with HIV are misled by anecdotal reports or by the exploitive marketing of nutritional products of unproven worth (or worse). While much basic research remains to be done, those gains we have made need to be drawn upon and put into action. Tragically, the information that *has* been laboriously accrued remains largely the exclusive domain of the medical/academic community and, like the tree falling in the abandoned forest, makes no meaningful sound. It is time to get this information into the hands of the people who need it, every day, to live! That is what *Cooking for Life* is about.

Cooking for Life draws on up-to-date research and gives both the background information and the rationale for sound nutritional practices. It also outlines dietary modifications necessary for addressing health problems that are intrinsically related to diet. Written by a chef, the information is delivered in a conversational, lay manner, accessible both to the sophisticated patient, and to the health professional, counselor, or case manager to whose lot it may fall to advise or consult the less educated patient. Above all, it is designed to be a practical reference of ongoing use through every stage of HIV disease. Nutrition is a vital component of health; for someone with HIV, nutritional intervention should begin at diagnosis.

Preface

When I was first interviewed to open the kitchen at the Metropolitan AIDS Neighborhood Nutrition Alliance (MANNA), nothing was asked or even mentioned concerning my knowledge of nutrition, and it was a good thing; though I had been cooking one way or another for more than twenty-five years, I had never paid more than cursory attention to nutrition. I could not have really explained the difference between a protein and a carbohydrate if someone had asked.

Quickly, I began to look around for nutrition information pertinent to HIV to add to my own slight knowledge. What I found was that there was nothing available geared to the lay reader except a score of slim pamphlets offering a superficial glance at the subject, all of which stressed the great importance of good nutrition. Understanding the available medical literature was, at the time, far beyond my reach.

As I began to accrue a body of practical information, I was fortunate enough to be put in touch with two experts in the field, Norma Muurahainen and Peggi Guenter, who would patiently instruct me and who gave unselfishly of their personal time as we three embarked upon offering a series of cooking/nutrition/food-safety classes for people living with HIV and their caregivers. It is one thing to tell people that they need more protein in their diet; another to tell them what it is and how to get it there: how to fry an egg.

Onto this information I was able to cobble insight born of personal experience. As a feckless college student I had strep throat that, before seeking medical advice, I allowed to progress to the point where I could barely swallow. Even swallowing milk was agony. Naturally thin to begin with, I struggled for nine months to regain the fifteen pounds I had lost during my illness. Ten years later I was in bed for a month with hepatitis, frequently overcome with nausea and growing weaker from enforced bed rest. Experiences that had seemed lamentable suddenly became tools for understanding.

Through these several years I was constantly amazed that this book did not exist. Leaving MANNA, I began to work on AmFAR-sponsored HIV/nutrition research, interviewing many individuals at every stage of HIV disease about their health, quality of life, and nutritional profiles. If I had any lingering doubt about the vital importance of good nutrition in the face of HIV, it was wiped away by that experience. I was often touched and instructed by the insights of thoughtful, caring individuals I encountered in this project. One of them was Margaret Cauterucci, my third adviser to this book.

I come to the issues of death and dying first through volunteering with hospice, later through a multitude of AIDS/service-organization involvements. It is a platitude to tell someone to live every day as though it is his or her last. To be confronted with our own mortality is something else altogether. But as surely as shadow gives form and definition to light, the bracket of death gives meaning to our lives. Those who face death are among the most vibrantly alive I have ever known and I am honored and privileged by their perspective. During the course of writing this book, I have lost a great favorite of my heart to HIV and my own mother has died. My connection to death has been far from merely organizational.

So this book is written to myself, five years ago, and to you. Don't be daunted by fears that the subject is too vast or difficult to learn. Don't be misled as to the value of its practical application. Don't fail to take care of yourself.

Nutrition and Long-Term Survival

Studies of long-term survivors of AIDS reveal five identifying characteristics:

1. Commitment to living
2. Active participation in one's own well-being
3. Flexibility
4. Long-term goals
5. Networking with other people with AIDS

Let's consider those five individually.

COMMITMENT TO LIVING: At a casual glance it is easy to assume that everyone desires to go on living. However, chronic illness and pain, as well as psychological and spiritual discouragement, can take their toll on all of us. Life is not the only choice. Some people choose not to fight to survive. But if living is our choice, we must steel our resolve to guard it against times when unpleasantness crowds our experience and seems to comprise it.

ACTIVE PARTICIPATION IN ONE'S OWN WELL-BEING: This means taking command and responsibility for your place and actions in life. It has been shown that the person who works in informed partnership with his physician stands to gain the most from the relationship. Ask questions. Don't passively relinquish control of your life. There are no absolutes, even in medicine. Disagreement is allowable.

It is the actively involved person who, when confronted with two options, will generally choose the one that is the more healthy for her. This does not necessarily mean a life of duty and asceticism. The soul needs to be fed as well. "Should I stay up late and play?" Only you can determine whether rest or relaxation is more beneficial at a given moment. This is not a license for self-indulgence, but rather encouragement to thoughtfully and holistically access your needs and take responsibility for meeting them.

FLEXIBILITY: This means a willingness to change to accommodate changing needs. Some people ask, "How can you say I should give up smoking, when it is one of the few pleasures I have left?" Emphatically, it is their right to smoke. But there are clear consequences to any action, and inflexibility of that kind does not contribute to long-term survival. These things are not moral issues but rather designs for living. Perhaps a less obvious example is the need to remove yourself from situations that are unduly stressful, such as a bad job or relationship. This book focuses on the changes you may need to make in your diet after the diagnosis of HIV. The fulfillment of your changing needs will buttress your survival.

LONG-TERM GOALS: We all need something to get out of bed for in the morning, some focus. Failing that, we lack resolve and drift. Why enroll in law school if you'll be dead in eighteen months? Because there is every reason to believe you *won't* be dead in eighteen months unless you hang on to that attitude. What if you're confined to bed? Ever read *War and Peace*? It is difficult to maintain a commitment to living when living has no definition. The achievement of the goal is secondary here (though by definition a goal must have meaning). The quest is the goal.

NETWORKING WITH OTHER PEOPLE WITH AIDS: No matter how great another's empathy, the old adage is true that no one can understand our situation until he has walked a mile in our shoes.

Feelings of isolation or connectedness determine our fundamental relationship to the human condition and this, in part, means finding commonality with our fellow human beings. Whether the common issues are a parent's alcoholism or the encroachments of middle age, comparing notes with someone in a similar situation to ourselves serves to diminish apprehension of the unknown. Failing that, we stand alone and abandoned by those whose insight, born of experience, might otherwise sustain us through unfamiliar circumstances.

Good nutrition embraces the first three of those five characteristics of long-term survivors! In fact, when paired with exercise, which provides complementary health benefits, it is hard to imagine an individual response to HIV that would be more life affirming.

Only a few years ago the cohort of long-term survivors of AIDS was widely considered statistically insignificant. Today, after seventeen years of tracking, some studies indicate that up to 33 percent of people with HIV are not only long-term survivors, but show no progression to AIDS. Though great advances in medical technology are part of this change, the contribution of improved nutritional awareness and practice cannot be overstated.

Martin Delaney, founding director of Project Inform*, says, "Beyond antiretrovirals or immune-system reconstruction or any other technological approach, good nutrition is the single greatest enhancement for the immune system." As we come into an era where our views of medicine and health are undergoing radical transformation, this awareness is only apt to grow. The time for nutritional intervention in your own life is now!

---

*Project Inform is a San Francisco–based organization that advocates for experimental drug trials and seeks to educate potential participants.

HOW TO USE THIS BOOK

People are remarkably different one from another, and not only in our diets and habits; our specific biological needs can vary enormously. Age and sex are two obvious factors; health status is another. Beyond that there is an individuality to our biological and metabolic functioning that is difficult at times to understand, much less to assess. Further, HIV is a disease that manifests itself in different people in ways varying from subtle to dramatic. Finally, each stage of HIV disease calls for a different strategy and response. This book is designed to help you sort through both the basic and the changing needs, and to meet the challenges; to give you information useful for crafting a long and healthy life for yourself. The information offered is not a directive, but is intended as a helpful guide that you may pick and choose from and tailor to your needs; variance from or adherence to suggested guidelines is a matter of personal choice. Responsibility for determining and staying the course will always devolve upon you. It is my hope that this book will better allow you to make your choices informed ones.

To begin you need a baseline of information and a team. Your team should start with your (AIDS-knowledgeable) physician, but should not end there. A knowledgeable pharmacist brings something to your health care quite different from what your physician brings; so does a nutritionist. None of these has the same expertise as an exercise therapist or a sensitive nurse, who may have many suggestions of ways to make your life qualitatively better. You may decide to add acupuncture, Chinese herbal medicine, or other nontraditional methods to your treatment regimen. Each of these has something unique to offer: this is your advisory panel, your team. You are the captain.

The first two parts of this book—"Nutrition and Exercise" and "Food and Water Safety"—contain elemental information that all of us need to live lives of optimal good health, symptomatic or not. Also, read in Part Three, the chapter entitled "Strategies for Weight Gain and Maintenance."

The title of Part Three is "Dietary Troubleshooting"; if you are currently experiencing any health problems related to food or diet, go straight to the appropriate chapter there.

If you know nothing of cooking, it would behoove you to learn some fundamentals, for that will allow you much greater control over your diet and limit your exposure to potentially dangerous food-poisoning pathogens. Part Four is designed to help with this. It presents information for the beginning and the experienced cook alike, in addition to suggestions for nutrition management (such as budget eating).

PART ONE

Nutrition
and Exercise

HIV and Wasting

Probably the single most vivid and frightening image of the impact of HIV on an individual is that of a gaunt, emaciated person whose grasp on life seems as fragile as his body. Wasting. Wasting is malnutrition, the body's inability to get or utilize the nutrients it needs to sustain itself. When malnutrition occurs, the body begins to rob from its stores of fat, protein, calcium; in short—to absorb itself.

Although wasting is the second most frequent AIDS-defining condition in the United States, **progressive wasting is not an invariable consequence of AIDS.** Wasting only results from specific causes. These causes can be psychological, such as despondency and lack of interest in food; physiological, such as parasitic infestation; mechanical, such as debilitating mouth or throat soreness; or simply financial, the inability to afford food. It is of paramount importance that efforts be made to discover and treat the underlying causes of wasting in any individual experiencing rampant weight loss. While this is not always so simple or straightforward as it may sound, survival itself, not to mention quality of life, may depend on determining and correcting the situation.

MALABSORPTION

In a healthy person the nutrients from foods are processed and absorbed at every stage of passage through the alimentary canal or "gut," which extends from the lips to the anus. Any compromise of this system, from loss of teeth to atrophy of the intestines, reduces its overall efficiency. Malabsorption is the inability of the body to process and utilize the food we eat despite its actual intake. It is what most people mean when they refer to "wasting" and, again, though it can occur for a number of reasons when the gut is damaged beyond its ability to function, there is no generalized malabsorption connected with AIDS. As with any wasting, malabsorption occurs only for a specific cause or causes such as amoebic infestation or chronic diarrhea and, with accurate early diagnosis, treatment, and luck, may be reversed. Any dramatic involuntary weight loss demands medical attention. However, malabsorption is an extreme medical condition whose cause can be difficult to diagnose and remedy. Far better to avoid the occurrence as much as possible by preventive measures (such as those discussed in Part Two, "Food and Water Safety"). If lack of intake or appropriate diet is deemed not to be the cause of weight loss, aggressive medical investigation to determine its origins is vital. Due to the difficulties of diagnosis, it is preferable to consult a gastroenterologist who makes a speciality of AIDS. Lacking this, it is important that your AIDS-knowledgeable physician be mindful of these problems and be up to date on diagnostic and treatment issues.

> **At any stage of AIDS, conservation of lean body mass is the central concern. The presence or lack of lean body mass is a more accurate predictor of survival than T-cell counts.**

LEAN BODY MASS*

By weight the human body is comprised of water, fat, skeletal weight, and protein matter, also known as "lean body mass" or "body cell mass." Lean body mass is composed of muscle, hair, nails, and all organ matter. When you do not get (or cannot absorb) from your food the protein your body needs, your system cannot replace those cells which are constantly wearing out (and which, under normal circumstances, are constantly replaced). To accomplish this necessary function your body must steal protein from that store of lean body mass which is least essential to its functioning—the muscle mass. If this situation continues for a long time, your body is then forced to turn to organ matter as an alternate source of protein. Thus the heart, liver, pancreas, and all of the body's organs are diminished.

As protein loss continues, our body's overall ability to function is compromised until any onslaught of infection is too great and our bodies succumb. In all situations, **even without the presence of HIV,** malnutrition is shown to increase rates of infection.

Research into the observations of starvation made by physicians in the Warsaw ghetto during World War II and of hunger strikers in Ireland in the 1970s show that even in otherwise healthy people, **the body cannot sustain life beyond the 30–33-percent loss of ideal lean body mass.** At that point the body simply cannot mount a successful defense to even the simplest attack. For example, an individual may have experienced repeated bouts of Pneumocystis carinii pneumonia (PCP), recovering each time but continuing to lose weight. At the point at which that person has lost one third of her lean body mass, another occurrence of PCP proves fatal. In each of the previous episodes the patient was able to withstand the attack to her health; the variation in this final chapter is malnutrition.

Looking at the matter from a slightly different perspective, **most deaths from AIDS are deaths of starvation.** Overall

* The more precise scientific term is *body cell mass,* which accounts for all the body's protoplasm. *Lean body mass* is the more common terminology and is used here for conversational ease.

BODY MASS INDEX

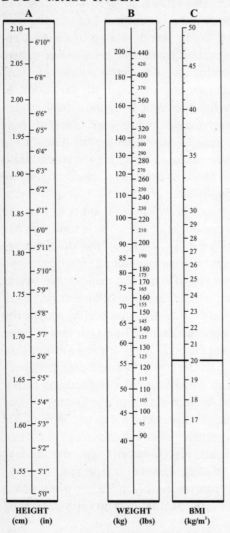

HEIGHT		WEIGHT		BMI
(cm)	(in)	(kg)	(lbs)	(kg/m²)

BODY MASS INDEX CALCULATOR

Body Mass Index (BMI) is a reflection of height and weight proportions. Though not a true determinant of lean body mass, it is a nonetheless helpful guide to a healthy weight range.

On the chart to the left:

1. Find your height on column A.

2. Find your weight on column B.

3. Using a straight-edge join the points on column A and B, extending the line to column C.

The point at which the line crosses column C is your BMI. It should be at least 20. If it is below that, aggressive measures should be made to increase your overall weight, stressing weight gain of lean body mass as described in chapters 1 through 4.

weight correlates only generally to lean body mass and therefore cannot be used as a reliable index. A former athlete who has become a "couch potato" might find that while he may weigh the same, all of his pants fit more tightly. Muscle, which is dense and heavy, has been converted to fat; therefore one could be overweight and still suffer from malnutrition. Loss of lean body mass in this manner is just as detrimental as any other.

DETERMINING BODY COMPOSITION

Lean body mass can only accurately be determined by using technical instruments designed for the purpose—instruments which, unfortunately, are not widely available. Your doctor may be able to implement such tests; alternatively, some health clubs maintain equipment to monitor the development of muscle in their members who are working out.

Most commonly available (and least accurate) are skinfold calipers, which measure the fat deposits in the skin in several places on the body along with bicep circumference. This test is acceptable, but its accuracy varies widely depending largely on the expertise of the person administering it. In many health clubs the training for this test is only cursory, and the level of accuracy correspondingly suspect. If the skinfold-calipers test is the only one available to you for checking your lean body mass (as it commonly is), the best plan is to have it performed at regular intervals—perhaps once a month—and take a running average of the totals. The point here is not to determine an absolute number, but to see in which direction you are moving, whether toward loss or gain.

Hydrodensitrometry (underwater weighing) assesses body composition by submersion/displacement in a saline solution and is a highly accurate technique of accessing percentage body fat. Because of the elaborate equipment and procedure involved, it is probably the least widely available method of testing. This system is found in some technically oriented sports training facilities and hospitals, especially those which specialize in weight-loss programs.

Bioelectrical impedance analysis (BIA) is another highly accurate method of determining lean body mass and one of rapidly growing availability. A BIA machine is a small device that measures body composition by sending minute and unfelt electrical charges through the body and analyzing the resistance at different frequencies. Because of its great accuracy and relatively low expense, it is gaining popularity in both the medical and health-club communities.

Should none of these tests be available to you, my first suggestion is to prevail upon an AIDS service organization in your area to provide them. At least expense, the skinfold calipers should be within the reach of almost any organization. Failing that, perhaps the group can arrange with a local health club or medical facility to provide testing as a service to its clients.

General observations about your own body can also provide you with clues. An unaccustomed leanness in your thighs, rump, or biceps indicates a loss of lean body mass. If your pants fit more tightly but your weight has remained the same, muscle has shifted to fat. Bulk may, however, be a result of water retention rather than increase of either fat or muscle, so it is not a completely reliable indicator.

METABOLISM AND EXERCISE

Basal metabolism is the rate at which our resting bodies use energy to maintain all basic functions. In times of energetic exercise the metabolic rate is increased and more energy is expended. Conversely, when we are lethargic, our rate of metabolism decreases, and we conserve energy. The body attempts to maintain homeostasis, or balance, so that the amounts of energy expended and stored are equal.

During times of infection, for each degree of fever our metabolism increases its energy needs by 7 percent, such is the increased demand on our immune system for action and response. To counterbalance this increase other metabolic processes are slowed. This is why we feel tired during times of sickness and why bed rest is recommended. This is also why it is of vital importance to maintain an adequate—which may mean increased—nutritional intake.

An important second phenomenon occurs whenever our rate of activity slows. As we become less active, our lean body mass converts from muscle to fat and we effectively lose lean body mass (even if our overall weight has remained the same). Furthermore, with the loss of muscle, we are apt to become increasingly sedentary and lethargic, thus creating a self-perpetuating syndrome of muscle loss/decreased metabolism/additional resulting muscle loss. Therefore safeguarding our muscle mass through exercise is of twofold importance. One of the most effective weapons in the fight against wasting is a regimen of weight-bearing exercise. This will be discussed at length in Chapter 4, "Exercise."

DETERMINING NUTRITIONAL INTAKE:
THE FOOD DIARY

All our lives are cluttered with habits we take so much for granted that we cease to notice them. Our habits of eating tend to be among these. If we are not especially hungry and take a few bites of a sandwich, we may feel that we have had lunch and think no more about it. Of course, there is a vast quantitative difference between a few bites of a sandwich and half of a roast chicken with vegetables and dessert, though six days later probably all we remember is that we haven't skipped lunch in at least a week.

Do not assume that you can rely solely on memory to analyze your own diet. Most people do not retain accurate memories of their food intake. For you, or for a dietary counselor, to accurately understand what you have been eating, it is necessary to keep a food diary. This can help you to discover the true causes of weight loss. What might be supposed to arise from malabsorption may instead be the result of diminished appetite or of filling up on foods with "incomplete" proteins or other "empty" calories.

Ideally a food diary not only records times when weight loss is a concern, but "normal" times as well, so that relative changes in diet may be gauged. On the following pages are blank diary sheets to fill in on a daily basis. Photocopy as many as you need. It should only take a few minutes each day to fill it in. This vital record of your food intake will help a dietary counselor or other health-care provider to assess crucial components of your diet which may be lacking and to structure appropriate modifications.

FOOD DIARY

Date _____   Weight _____

Time	Meal	Food Eaten	Amount
_____	Breakfast		
_____	Snack		
_____	Lunch		
_____	Snack		
_____	Dinner		
_____	Snack		

Medications: _____   Times taken: _____

_____

_____

_____

_____

Exercise: _____   Time spent: _____

Vitamin Supplements: _____

Appetite: *Excellent*   *Good*   *Fair*   *Poor*

Breakfast   _____

Lunch   _____

Dinner   _____

Digestive Upsets:

Symptoms: _____

Times: _____

Comments*: _____

_____

_____

_____

_____

* Examples: ate home/ate out; with company/alone; appetite great, food terrible; missed lunch because of meeting, slept well/slept poorly, etc.

FOOD DIARY

Date _____   Weight _____

Time	Meal	Food Eaten	Amount
_____	Breakfast	_____	
_____	Snack	_____	
_____	Lunch	_____	
_____	Snack	_____	
_____	Dinner	_____	
_____	Snack	_____	

Medications: _____   Times taken: _____

_____

_____

_____

_____

_____

Exercise: _____   Time spent: _____

Vitamin Supplements: _____

Appetite: *Excellent*   *Good*   *Fair*   *Poor*

Breakfast   _____

Lunch   _____

Dinner   _____

Digestive Upsets:

Symptoms: _____

Times: _____

Comments*: _____

_____

_____

_____

_____

_____

* Examples: ate home/ate out; with company/alone; appetite great, food terrible; missed lunch because of meeting, slept well/slept poorly, etc.

Basic Nutrition

Though models of good nutrition come and go, perhaps the most unchanging and "bottom line" statement that can be made of a healthy diet is that it should be wide ranging. This also presupposes moderation in any single dietary direction. For example, if broccoli is your only vegetable, chances are that you will be missing out on any number of trace elements and micronutrients found in other vegetables. While nutritional research can be said to be in more than its infancy, it is not much past childhood as a scientific discipline. Essential dietary components, heretofore unknown, are still constantly being discovered. Latest of these to gain widespread attention in the media are "phytochemicals," a vast family of chemical compounds abundant in plant source foods (fruits and vegetables) that are grown in sunlight. Although it appears that phytochemicals have important cancer-fighting properties, the very category was unknown five years ago and cataloging of them has only just begun. No single group of foods or vitamin/mineral supplements can hope to assure sufficiency in this or any other category of vital nutrients we know of, much less those categories still waiting to be identified. Therefore, the more wide ranging a diet, the greater the assurance that no deficiency will occur.

The foods we eat can be cast into several models of nutrition, some of the models better than others, none perfect. Several generations of Americans have grown up thinking that eggs are a dairy product because in the old "Four Food Groups" model, where did they go? They clearly weren't grains or vegetables, and though they are animal protein, they weren't meat or fish. Since the long-gone milkman delivered them, they must be dairy. But if far more than half the world's population never sees milk beyond mother's milk, can this group really be said to be an essential food group?

The current model of nutrition is the Food Pyramid, which basically shuffles the Four Food Groups deck slightly and prioritizes its components (with a P.S. capstone to let us know that we shouldn't eat too much fat or oils). Canada styles this the "Food Rainbow." Both models are designed to indicate the best proportions of various types of food in an ideal diet. While these models are a fair depiction of typical needs, a more thorough understand-

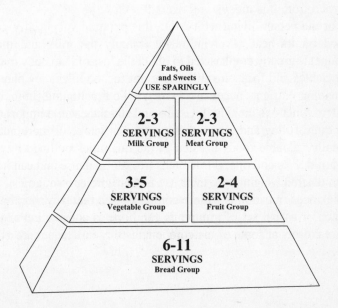

ing of what we derive from these categories is essential to our making effective use of the information.

The portions listed above may seem like an enormous amount of food for one person to eat in a single day until you realize that Those Who Know Best are very stingy. One slice of bread is considered a serving, so that a sandwich constitutes two servings of grain. A small glass of juice is a serving of fruit. One cup of lettuce is a serving of vegetable. (Now really, put one cup of lettuce on a plate and ask yourself if that could possibly be considered a salad in even a very chic restaurant. These people could stretch a Thanksgiving turkey to feed forty people!)

For the asymptomatic HIV-positive person the *proportions* of foods as organized by the Food Pyramid are not a bad reference. As a portion-*counting* system, however, it makes slight allowance for body size, age, sex, or activity level. Counting portions this way, a three-egg omelet (eggs are now in the meat group) is a total day's meat-group serving for stevedores and diminutive grandmothers alike. Relative proportions of foods are what may best be learned from this model.

For the person living with AIDS this pyramid very nearly gets stood on its head. Protein intake (mainly the milk and meat groups) is greatly emphasized to offset the loss of lean body mass. Vegetables and fruits are still important for the roles they play in providing nutrients necessary to metabolic functioning (immune-system functions included). Grains and starches, while important, are quite filling and may therefore prevent intake of more nutritionally valuable foods if eaten in the quantities outlined by the pyramid. Fats and oils, if tolerated, are calorie dense and can help with desired weight gain; their use is therefore encouraged.

Balanced nutrition is a more complex issue than any thumbnail sketch or casual set of groupings can hope to convey. Let's look more closely at some of the components these models represent.

CALORIES

What is a calorie? A calorie is a measure of energy. To be exact, it is the amount of energy it takes to raise one gram of water one degree centigrade. Calories are also the measure of the energy that fuels our bodies. In terms of nutrition some calories are more valuable than others, not because they contain more energy than other calories (again, a calorie is simply a unit measuring that energy), but because of what else may come packaged with them. For example, alcohol and refined sugars contain calories, but no additional nutrients. Such calories are referred to as "empty calories"; they do provide the body with energy, but nothing else, making them a very poor nutritional bargain. On the other hand, the calories in meat or vegetables contain a wealth of nutrients, such as protein, vitamins, and minerals, all of which are essential to healthy body functioning. If we take in more calories than we utilize, our bodies store the extra as fat. The best idea, of course, is to make all of our caloric intake as valuable as possible and not to rely on excess caloric intake to assure we meet our nutritional needs.

CARBOHYDRATES

Virtually all the foods we eat have caloric value and all calories can be used by the body for its energy needs. However, the body's preferred and most readily usable source of energy comes to us from carbohydrates: sugars and starches that are converted by the body into sugars. Grains, such as wheat and rice, and "starchy" vegetables, such as potatoes, are our primary sources of carbohydrates, though many, many other foods contain them in much smaller quantities. For this reason carbohydrates (in their ideal form—grains, potatoes, and legumes) comprise the large base of the Pyramid.

Though "sweets" and alcohol are both carbohydrates, they are among the emptiest of calories. Do not be fooled by a nutritional label indicating that a soft drink or candy bar provides you with a stated percentage of your daily carbohydrates. These count for very little, if anything, nutritionally, save mere caloric intake itself. In great and constant quantities they can cause problems with the body's ability to metabolize sugars, not to mention offsetting the intake of more nutritious and valuable calories.

VITAMINS, MINERALS, TRACE ELEMENTS, AND MICRONUTRIENTS

What we don't know about vitamins can and undoubtedly will fill a book; many of them. As astonishing as it may seem, we really don't know exactly how vitamins function in the body. Most of our knowledge comes from observing what happens during specific vitamin deficiencies and making correlations. Unlike drug studies, where the potential profits of a successful patented drug are vast and pharmaceutical companies can therefore underwrite extensive research, no one has exclusive rights to vitamins and so the profit motive does not exist to drive important nutritional research.

Vitamins supply the body with chemical compounds necessary for all its intricate biochemical functioning, including the immune system. *Vita* is Latin for "life." As their name implies, vitamins are not only essential to life, but are also derived from it; vitamins are organic substances (which can be synthesized chemically). Along with minerals they are required components of adequate nutrition and are supplied in our diets largely through our intake of fruits and vegetables. Beyond vitamins and minerals lies a vast category of nutrients, including trace elements, micronutrients, and phytochemicals. Many of these categories have only begun to be recognized and defined. Others doubtless are waiting to be discovered. Our understanding of their contributions to health lags far behind. For example, as mentioned above, researchers suspect that phytochemicals (specific nutrients abundant only in vegetables grown in sunlight) have important cancer-fighting properties. But because so little research has been conducted, we don't know if perhaps it is simply that a diet rich in phytochemicals is also rich in fiber and to that should be attributed its anticancer properties; or whether perhaps someone sated by a diet rich in fruits and vegetables simply doesn't eat much meat. What is known is that no pill can attempt to match the array of essential nutrients supplied by eating a variety of fruits and vegetables.

Recommended Dietary Allowances, determined by the Food and Nutrition Board of the National Academy of Sciences–National Research Council, are *very* general guidelines only. Common sense will tell you that a 110-pound menopausal female with a desk job and a 240-pound twenty-seven-year-old male professional athlete will have vastly differing vitamin needs, though the RDA is the same for them both. Add variables such as stress or smoking, which deplete nutrients from the body, and most guidelines begin to lose all proportion.

Vitamin pills are supplements, not substitutes, for regular dietary intake. With anything approaching a normal diet it is unlikely that you will overdo your vitamin intake, but with supplements the questions arise, "How much is good? How much more is better? How much is too much?" Many people like to play mix and match with vitamin supplements, often multiplying the RDAs many times over. For example, hearing that zinc is necessary for immune-system functioning, some people will gulp zinc supplements like popcorn. Too much zinc, however, can interfere with the body's copper absorption, causing problems equal to or exceeding those potentially caused by a slight lack of zinc. Since vitamins function synergistically, a balance of vitamins and minerals is what is needed and appropriate. The easiest way to achieve this is to use a wide-spectrum multivitamin with mineral supplement (such as Centrum). Since even slight malabsorption can offset this intake in people living with HIV, it is recommended to take two such tablets a day, one in the morning and one in the evening. By doing this you are assured of a benign excess of vitamins and minerals, but not an imbalance or toxic excess.

The price of vitamins is not an index of quality. Study after study shows that nutritive value and the efficiency and rate of absorption are not related to the price of various brands of vitamins. In fact, sometimes the reverse is true. Vitamins from health-food

stores are no better than those from the discount shelf in your local drugstore. Generic versions of name brands are by far your
best bargain and are absolutely just as good.

For most people absorption is optimized if vitamins are taken
before a meal, but if vitamin tablets give you indigestion, try taking them during or after meals.

To conclude: A slice of toast and a vitamin pill is not a good
breakfast. A hot dog and a vitamin pill is not a good lunch. A slice
of pizza and a vitamin pill is not a good dinner. Good nutrition can
only come from eating a balanced diet. The vastly complex needs
of our bodies can only be met by a wide range of foods supplying
compounds as yet undreamt of by scientists, much less included
in any pill.

PROTEIN

Protein is the substance of the body's lean mass (our organs and
our muscle) and, for purposes of human consumption, is composed of twenty-two building blocks called amino acids, all of
which are necessary if the human body is to use any of them. To
have a truckload of twenty of the necessary amino acids and none
of the remaining two is, in terms of nutrition, virtually the same
as having none at all. For this reason foods containing all of the
necessary amino acids are commonly referred to as "complete
proteins." Complete proteins are readily available to us from animal food sources only: meat, poultry, fish, eggs, and dairy products, with the latter two being the forms most efficiently used by
the body.* In all cases these foods supply us with every single one
of the amino acids necessary to meet our body's protein needs.

Protein is also abundantly available to us from plant matter, but
in an "incomplete" form. Though many plant-based foods offer a

* Gelatin and egg whites are the sole exceptions to the rule that all animal-source proteins
provide complete proteins. For this reason egg substitutes, such as Egg Beaters (which are
composed solely of egg whites) should *not* be counted upon to supply complete proteins,
though their incomplete proteins may combine with others in the diet to form complementary proteins.

great deal of protein, no single vegetable matter offers a full complement of the necessary twenty-two amino acids. We therefore must be careful to balance one vegetable food with others which will supply those amino acids lacking from the first, thereby forming a "complementary protein." This is another reason to eat a variety of foods every day.

The vast majority of the world gets its protein from plant-based foods, and this is the most economical way. Every culture has devised indigenous dishes that supply this complement: red beans and rice are a classic example. Corn tortillas and refried beans are another. There is an easy rule that makes determining the bulk of these combinations simple. **Any combination of a legume* with grains, sesame seeds, or nuts (with the exception of cashews) will create a complementary protein.**

For example: a peanut-butter sandwich. The protein from peanuts (which are a legume) combines with the complementary protein from bread (the grain wheat) to form a complete protein that fuels the growth of so many ever-taller adolescents in this country. Proteins that complement one another do not need to be eaten in the same dish or even necessarily in the same meal. Any bean/legume and grain complementation eaten within about an hour of one another will combine in the body to form a complete protein. For a recipe for a flour formula that is a complete protein, see "Enriched Flour" on page 176.

Another way to take advantage of the abundant and economical protein offered by vegetable sources is to supply their missing complement of amino acids with minute amounts of animal protein. Rice, the great foodstuff and protein source of much of the world's population, is by itself an incomplete protein. However, even a few shreds of pork, as in so much native Chinese cuisine, will supply in abundance the amino acids missing from the rice.

* Legumes include black beans, black-eyed peas, chickpeas, kidney beans, lentils, lima beans, mung beans, navy beans, peanuts, pinto beans, red beans, split peas, and soybeans. For suggestions on how to cook legumes, see recipe on page 165. Grains include barley, buckwheat, corn, oats, rice, rye, and wheat.

The body is by this means able to utilize the substantial amounts of protein in the rice that would otherwise be useless to it. This complementary relationship is true of all vegetable and animal protein combinations (including dairy and egg sources), as animal proteins are laden with those amino acids commonly missing from vegetable-matter proteins.

Your body's daily need for protein is not actually large. If cooked meat were your *only* source of protein (a situation not likely to occur in any diet remotely approaching normal), approximately a seven-ounce portion would supply all that an average adult needs. However, virtually any diet, even one heavy in meat, also includes protein from other sources (dairy products, complementary vegetable proteins, and so on) beyond average needs. What is essential is an intake of complete protein every day to repair and replace the millions of cells that are constantly wearing out. Should your diet fail to supply this, your body will be forced to rob from its stores of protein (your muscle mass) in order to fulfill this need.

Contrary to their ability to store fat, our bodies have no efficient methods for storing protein. Anything above and beyond our basic daily need is simply excreted in the urine and does no good whatsoever. In fact, chronic bingeing on protein can unduly tax the kidneys and cause problems of its own. This most often happens when people, recognizing the importance of protein in their diet, use "weight gain" products designed for the increased needs of competition body builders. These products can cause other problems as well, including diarrhea. As stated elsewhere, there is no magic "food pill" or other substitute for real food. Remember: Seven ounces of cooked meat is a very small portion, not to mention the protein you get from sources besides meat.

FATS AND OILS

Fats and oils tend to have bad press these days for the good reason that the typical American diet is much too heavy in these calorie-dense food sources (as we all have been told, again and again). What is seldom said is that these components of diet are necessary, both because fat-soluble vitamins (A, D, E, and K) are only utilized by the body in the context of fats and because of the body's need for *essential fatty acids*. Some fats are more nutritionally valuable than others.

Essential fatty acids are found primarily in polyunsaturated oils and are necessary to all of the body's cell structure. Corn oil, sunflower oil, soy oil, linseed oil, safflower oil, and wheat-germ oil are all excellent sources of essential fatty acids. Olive and canola oils are not good sources of these important ingredients. In all but the most fat-restricted diet you should have no problem getting sufficient fat intake. However, should your fat intake be severely restricted (as in times of severe diarrhea), one teaspoon of the above recommended oils daily will assure adequate essential fatty acids.

Looking back at the Food Pyramid, you can see that proteins, vitamins, minerals, and fats may be found in all categories, though in differing quantities and concentrations. Very generally, in a sort of dietary shorthand, it can be said that:

• Calories, by themselves, are the measure of fuel on which the body runs.

• Carbohydrates (grains, potatoes, rice, and sugars) supply the body with sustained fuel.

• Vitamins, minerals, trace elements, and micronutrients (fruits and vegetables) supply the vast and complex components needed to facilitate the chemical functioning of the body (immune functions included).

• Proteins (meats, eggs, dairy products, complementary vegetable proteins) supply material with which to build the body in childhood and rebuild it from ongoing wear and tear.

• Fats and oils, in a balanced diet, supply us about 30 percent of our caloric intake. They also provide us with essential fatty acids, necessary to all body cell structure.

The same foods frequently come to us in many different forms. Green beans, for example, many be purchased fresh, frozen, or canned. The same food may also come to us in differing degrees of "refinement," such as whole wheat flour versus unbleached flour versus bleached flour. How to choose the most nutritious of these various forms?

In the case of degrees of refinement, the choice is simple: the less a food is refined, the more it retains its natural nutritional value. (The "added" value in chemically fortified and enriched foods refers more to vitamin and mineral supplements than to genuine foodstuffs. Some processed breakfast cereals contain more sugar by percentage weight than a chocolate bar, but, because they are fortified and enriched, tout themselves as nutritious.) A simple illustration of the greater value of less refined food is to compare the nutritional labels of "plain" and whole wheat versions of the same brand of a product such as an English muffin. You can easily see that the whole wheat has greater protein value. In a thorough nutritional analysis, many more advantages would be apparent. This advantage holds true for all less refined foodstuffs. The exception to this rule for people living with HIV is that if the digestive tract is in a fragile state, some less refined foods (for example, brown rice versus white rice) can contribute to motility and, if diarrhea is present, are best avoided. For a complete discussion of fiber issues, refer to Chapter 10.

In the case of fresh, frozen, canned, or dried options, the case is less clear. Generally, a fresh vegetable would be the ideal nutritional choice, but if it is withered and shriveled and fresh only by virtue of not being cooked, canned, frozen, or dried, it is certainly not likely to retain much nutritive value. Much better would be a vegetable flash-frozen at its peak of freshness. Even proper canning (with minimal processing and additives) is more likely to preserve food value. A hard, green winter tomato is unlikely to match a tomato canned at prime summer ripeness in either taste or nutrition. Certain foods, such as legumes, suffer virtually no nutritional loss from being canned or dried. The goal is to obtain prime foods held at that prime through the least amount of processing necessary. This is largely determined by the length of time a food is to be preserved. Refrigeration works extremely well in most cases, but for short periods of time. Freezing is an excellent method of longer preservation, but at the expense of cell-membrane disruption, which contributes to moisture loss. Canning is suitable for even longer-term preservation, but the high heats required cause much vitamin loss. Another method is chemical preservatives (largely antibacterial agents), which are much less desirable.

In all of the above-mentioned cases the object is to select food as near as possible to its ideal natural state—frozen green beans that are crisp and green, not canned ones that are limp and gray.

Somewhere in these pages you, the reader, are apt to see the error of your dastardly ways and be tempted to a repentance and conversion of the tent-revival variety. Don't! This is why "diets" fail. Very, very few people are willing or able to throw out a lifetime of tastes and habits in one fell swoop and undertake a rigid new discipline without backsliding. This perceived failure then becomes reason to justify to ourselves why the whole project is unfeasible, especially if it is something we had mixed feelings about to begin with. The *New York Times* nutrition writer Jane Brody suggests "evolution, not revolution." Better to modify our habits so that we can live with the change and to strive constantly to improve by increments.

Special Nutritional Considerations for HIV+ Individuals

All of the basic tenets of sound nutrition as outlined in Chapter 2 hold true in light of HIV disease, though there is a shift in emphasis. Primarily, this emphasis is on protein intake. To ensure its adequacy, not only must the protein source be of sufficient quantity, but also of the right sort.

PROTEIN

If your appetite is diminished or your ability to eat is severely compromised, it is wise to focus on the protein portion of your meal. At such times it is the most vital component of your diet. Being mindful which foods provide complete or complementary proteins (see page 18), choose these protein foods first before filling up on other, less necessary items. For example: With a meal of meat loaf, mashed potatoes, and broccoli, many people, not feeling well, would head straight for the comfort food—mashed potatoes. The danger here is of filling up before getting around to the protein portion of the meal. If your appetite is slight, it's better to polish off the meat loaf first and then consider what else you may have room for. To repeat: You do not ever need a large protein intake at any one time, but you do need a daily intake of complete or complementary proteins. (See Chapter 1, "HIV and Wasting.")

CHOLESTEROL

Many of the standard cautions of diet go out the window in regard to HIV. Unless you have a preexisting condition of *extremely* high cholesterol, this should not be of concern to you. In fact, in the advance of HIV disease the tendency is for cholesterol to be stripped from the circulatory system. Since many calorie-laden high-protein foods, such as meat, cheese, and eggs, are also typically high in cholesterol, avoidance of those foods would severely restrict many of your most ready sources of protein and nutritiously valuable calories. More important by far is maintaining your weight and lean body mass.

SALT

Hypertension is another condition not typically associated with AIDS. If salting your food enhances your enjoyment of it and thereby improves your appetite, by all means do so. For someone with HIV disease, maintaining a healthy diet does not necessarily mean restricting salt intake. If, however, you suffer a preexisting or independent problem requiring salt restriction, you should follow the advice of your health-care provider.

DIET FADS

Nutrition is a national obsession. It is said that the only casual social comment as safe as the weather ("Hot enough for you?") is one about diet and nutrition. This was not always so. As *New York Times* health columnist Jane Brody points out, diet and nutrition were such "dead" topics only a few years back that even nutrition guru Adelle Davis wasn't able to use those very words in the titles of her books. Now, everybody loves to talk about diets, and with their popularity have come dozens of unsubstantiated fads. Enthusiastic anecdotal reports appear claiming miraculous gains in health. All too often such dietary regimens fly in the face of all known and substantiated nutritional logic and thus rob many people of a clear and proven course of diet. The reader is urged to carefully consider any unconventional dietary routine to determine whether or not it provides the known components necessary for all nutritional and metabolic needs. Beware of any food or diet that promises a panacea of health.

MACROBIOTICS

Some people will no doubt be surprised to find that this entire book is not devoted to the subject of the macrobiotic diet, as it is perceived by many to be extremely healthy and an antidote for all that is wrong with the typical American diet.

At the risk of making a controversial statement: you could hardly design a worse diet than macrobiotics for a person in any advanced stage of HIV disease, for three very important reasons. First, a macrobiotic diet is precariously low in protein, the issue of paramount concern. Second, it is extremely high in insoluble fiber, which can ravage an already delicate digestive tract. We will explore the topic of fiber in greater detail in Chapter 10. Third and finally, its practice is a very demanding discipline that requires almost daily shopping for fresh ingredients and substantial kitchen preparation several times a day, this last being hardly the expenditure of energy a sick person is apt to be willing or able to keep up with. Add to this the greater expense of organic produce, and you come up with a diet that undermines a person with AIDS on many levels.

This book attempts to offer the rationale for the components of a sound diet. It is up to you to decide if macrobiotics or any other diet assures adequate nutrition.

VEGETARIANISM

There are many misguided notions about vegetarianism, both pro and con. If you are a vegetarian or are considering becoming one, you will need to think carefully. Rigorous discipline is essential to adequate nutrition.

Without question it is possible to maintain a perfectly healthy diet from plant-food sources only. However, this is not likely to happen if you approach your diet in a random and haphazard manner. And a vegetarian diet does present some nutritional challenges.

To begin with, let's consider the general categories or varieties of vegetarianism, for the distinctions are important nutritionally. A total vegetarian is referred to as a "vegan" and eats no foods of animal origin whatsoever. A "strict" vegetarian (or ovolactovegetarian) may eat dairy products and eggs, but no "flesh." Many others who consider themselves vegetarians eat not only dairy and eggs, but also fish. Still others delete red meat from their diets, eating poultry as well as fish. These distinctions are nutritionally important, as we will see below.

First, there is no evidence that a vegan diet is healthier than one which includes small amounts of meat and other animal-source foods. Famously, the greatest concern for vegetarians is adequate protein intake, as the careful balancing of complementary proteins is necessary if the body is to find nourishment in plant food-stuffs (see page 19). Actually this concern is not the greatest challenge facing the typical vegetarian, though the issue becomes crucial to HIV-positive individuals, whose protein intake is a much more critical matter.

Many nutrients in plants (in addition to "incomplete" proteins) exist in a form that is very difficult or impossible for our bodies to use if not accompanied by other nutrients of a sort most commonly found in animal-source foods. For example, spinach is an excellent source of iron but presents it in a form largely unassimilable to someone who is a vegan. Roughly a truckload of spinach would have to be consumed **daily** to assure adequacy if this were your only source of iron. But with the concurrent intake of meat, the iron in spinach is accessible and readily utilized by the body. Another concern for vegans is adequate vitamin B_{12}, which is a necessary nutrient available to us only through animal sources or synthesized as a supplement. As many people with HIV tend to deficiency in B_{12}, its adequate intake is of great concern. Fortified nutritional yeast (NOT brewer's or baker's yeast), fortified soy milk, and vitamin B_{12} supplements are all possible alternative sources. Since there is some doubt whether B_{12} tablets are absorbed efficiently in the intestinal tract, alternative methods of delivery are constantly being developed. These include injection, sublingual (under-the-tongue) microdots, and nasal inhalants. Your health-care provider can monitor your B_{12} levels through routine blood work and recommend appropriate supplementation if needed.

With the addition of egg and dairy products to the diet, concerns for balanced and adequate nutrition loosen up. They are both widely known as "perfect foods" for the wide range of nutrients they provide in a very assimilable form. They also contain components which complement and make otherwise unusable plant-source nutrients available to our bodies. With cholesterol removed as a worry in the case of HIV, they become extremely valuable components of the diet and are a bargain, to boot.

Attention must be paid to overall caloric intake. Any vegetarian diet is apt to be low in calories, and this is doubly cause for concern for those with HIV. First, adequate caloric intake is of paramount importance to offset any involuntary weight loss. Second, if caloric intake is only marginally sufficient, protein calories may be burned to provide energy needs and protein reserves in the body will thus be jeopardized. To reemphasize, since the loss of lean body mass is an area of great concern to anyone who is HIV positive, it must always be guarded against.

Many people are vegetarian out of philosophical, not health, concerns. From the single viewpoint of nutrition, someone with HIV is well advised to incorporate animal protein into her diet. Nutrition, however, is not the sole consideration in any holistic view of health, much less of life, so each individual who grapples with this question must come to her own conclusion. If I may offer my personal perspective (as one who both shares my life with a fifteen-year-old dog—a cherished companion—

and who sits on the board of an animal refuge, such is my commitment to the humane and ethical treatment of animals), it is that eating meat is a sacred trust, not to be indulged in mindlessly or capriciously, but which is part of a natural chain of being. The other example I would offer is a story movingly told by Vivica Kraak, founding dietitian at God's Love We Deliver (New York's meal delivery program for people with AIDS). Years ago, Vivica, a vegetarian at the time, underwent extended hospitalization due to active tuberculosis. Able to read her own blood work, she could observe that the levels of albumin in her blood (a measure of the body's absorption of protein) were inadequate and did not respond to various modifications in diet. Since animal proteins are the highest-quality and most readily absorbed proteins, she made the decision to temporarily give up being a vegetarian so that she could nutritionally rebuild herself and not fall farther into malnutrition. Though Vivica is not HIV+, I include this story because it is an excellent example of the quality of flexibility, as described in the Introduction as one of the five necessary and identifying characteristics of long-term survivors of AIDS.

VITAMIN SUPPLEMENTS

As has been stated before, vitamin supplements are not substitutes for the regular, adequate dietary intake of foods abundant in vitamins and minerals—largely fruits and vegetables. To assure adequacy and err on the side of benign excess, a widespread multivitamin with mineral supplement taken morning and evening is recommended. Any brand that provides 100 percent of RDAs will do: Centrum or its generic counterpart—it's all the same to your body. Only your pocketbook will know the difference.

Vitamin B_{12} is the notable exception in vitamin needs as regards HIV. For reasons not understood, it is either malabsorbed or needed in much greater than normal quantities (possibly because of the characteristics of HIV itself, perhaps due to drug therapies). At any rate, should you be found, by your doctor or through blood work, to be vitamin B_{12} deficient, the remedy would be B_{12} injections, a B_{12} nasal inhalant, or sublingual microdot—not oral supplements, whose efficacy is uncertain.

ANTIOXIDANTS

Antioxidants, primarily the vitamins C, E, and the provitamin beta carotene, may also be required in greater quantity due to HIV. Rust, burning, and the deteriorating process of bleaching are all forms of oxidation. Oxidation is part of the aging process and is responsible for much of the wear and tear on our bodies as we grow older. During times of infection our bodies produce what are called "free oxygen radicals" in abundance as part of the body's immune response. These unstable molecules seek to latch their extra oxygen atom on to an invading bacterium, thereby oxidizing and destroying it. However, these molecules latch on to a great deal more than just bacteria; they latch on to you! During times of chronic infection, such as is common with HIV, the body produces such a constant stream of free oxygen radicals that there is undue wear and stress placed on it.

Antioxidants are substances that free oxygen radicals like to grab on to even more than they like grabbing on to you, and attached to which they are then harmlessly passed from the system. Some research suggests that antioxidants might help in this way to reduce the effects of aging. Vitamins C, E, and the provitamin beta carotene are the most notable antioxidants commonly found in foods. Also used is N-Acetyl-1-Cysteine (NAC), an antioxidant supplement (neither a necessary nutrient nor a drug), which is a potent antioxidant whose use has widespread endorsement in the HIV/medical community. It may be found in the vitamin section of many drugstores and most health-food stores and is typically taken at the rate of 600 mg three times a day.

Exercise

Western medicine has always been practiced as a healing rather than as preventative-maintenance art; consequently, nutrition and exercise have in general been given short shrift by the medical community. A little over a decade ago barely a medical school in the country required even a single course in nutrition of its students. Things have finally begun to change a little, in part because of the recognized impact of nutrition on those with HIV. The role of "second-class citizen" has been inherited by exercise. Though everyone agrees (as formerly with nutrition) that exercise is an important component to good health, most primary-care physicians receive little or no training on how to supervise exercise regimens for patients. This does *not,* however, mean that it is not an issue of vital importance. In terms of HIV, exercise can help in building stores of lean body mass and may also impact positively on immune-system functioning.

Exercise can be divided into two major types: aerobic and anaerobic (also called "weight-bearing" or "weight-resistance" training), both with their unique advantages.

AEROBIC EXERCISE

Aerobic exercise is any activity that utilizes the major muscle groups in a steady, rhythmical motion such as bicycling, jogging, or swimming. The primary goal of aerobic exercise is to strengthen the cardiovascular system. It also helps maintain smooth metabolic functioning and can help reduce stress and minimize depression. Preliminary research also indicates that aerobic exercise may stimulate T-cell production. Aerobic exercise does not build much muscle and does tend to strip fat from the body. Unless you're genuinely obese, weight loss should not be your goal in exercise. For that reason anaerobic (weight-bearing) exercise is generally a more valuable pursuit.

ANAEROBIC EXERCISE

In contrast to our efficient ability to store fat, the single way that our bodies hold extra lean body mass in reserve (or "stores protein") is in the form of extra muscle mass, which is developed only through a regimen of weight-resistance exercise. Because of the crucial importance of lean body mass, a weight-training exercise program is *strongly* recommended. This is possible at virtually any level of health or sickness. The weight you work with might be slight, but it will still help to maintain the integrity of the body's muscle mass. If you want to put "money in the bank of health," try working out regularly to build up some extra muscle as a hedge and buffer against a day when you may possibly need an extra store of lean body mass.

A good example of the different goals to be achieved by different routines of exercise is to look at how weight/repetition affects development. Fewer repetitions of higher weights result in larger, softer muscles. More repetitions at lower weights result in more defined (chiseled), harder muscles. This is because of an aerobic effect caused by the greater number of repetitions removing fat from the muscle, making it denser, more compact. Though fat is of comparatively little advantage, it does offer some counterbalance to involuntary weight loss. Again, working to remove fat is not the goal here. Structure your routine with an eye toward building rather than defining mass.

Ideally, a medically trained exercise therapist should design and monitor your routine; this category includes licensed physical therapists and exercise physiologists certified by the American College of Sports Medicine. If one is not available, do not, however, allow some marginally trained but enthusiastic gym-bunny (who in all likelihood is working off his own bartered club membership) to design an overly ambitious regimen for you. It is better to work slowly but steadily toward your goals. A realistic (versus ambitious) exercise program is important for a couple of reasons. First, you could hurt yourself. Do not feel shy about starting with weights that are quite low and working upward rather than risk injury by attempting too much too soon. Second, as with traditional dieting for weight loss, the greatest cause of failure is setting unrealistic goals and subsequently giving up in disillusionment. Having an exercise partner greatly helps in establishing and maintaining any exercise routine.

Finally, one of the most important aspects of regular exercise is that it promotes active participation in your own well-being—another of the identifying characteristics of long-term survivors of AIDS.

PART TWO

Food and Water Safety

Food Poisoning

It is estimated that 70 percent of all "twenty-four-hour flus" and gastrointestinal upsets that occur in this country are actually mild cases of food poisoning. Those who live with AIDS are seven times more susceptible to food-borne illness. Food poisoning, which may cause mild to severe discomfort in the general population, can prove lethal to those who are immunocompromised. Severe diarrhea is a primary symptom of most forms of food poisoning (see charts on pages 38 and 39). It is, along with vomiting, part of your body's defense mechanism to flush from itself the infectious agent. Either can lead to dehydration and rampant weight loss. Unfortunately, in many cases the pathogen is not entirely expelled by these means and the diarrhea can then become chronic and dangerous, fostering wasting. For these reasons food safety should be a conscious concern of all HIV-positive people. To circumvent or minimize the occurrence of poisoning, it is necessary both to maintain good food-handling practices and to work in tandem with your physician should an incident of suspected food poisoning arise.

Food poisoning is the result of naturally occurring pathogens that are harbored in many of our foodstuffs. These include bacteria, viruses, and microorganisms, such as parasitic amoebic infestations. Their presence, though difficult or impossible to detect by smell, taste, or appearance, is virulent and is the original and still the main reason that we cook many of our foods. Less virulent, but still capable of producing toxic reactions, are the funguses, yeasts, and bacteria that produce the more familiar food spoilage, with its telltale signs of odor and mold. The other great difference between food-spoilage organisms and food-poisoning organisms is that while the latter thrive at room temperature, their growth is retarded by low temperatures (hence the value and importance of prompt and adequate refrigeration). Food-spoilage organisms continue to multiply at temperatures even below 40 degrees.

Fifty years ago, only three agents of food poisoning were recognized; today, over twenty. In their ambience it is impossible to escape them. Rather, it is important to minimize our exposure by taking intelligent precautions. The quantity of a pathogen to which we are exposed, as well as the virulence of a particular strain, are both factors in determining the assault our immune systems face. However, as all pathogens can multiply rapidly in the right combination of warmth, moisture, and darkness, even a small amount of a given infectious agent may grow into a major problem. Additionally, immune systems of differing strengths can withstand varying degrees of onslaught.

The chart below lists the major types of food-borne pathogens that provide the greatest threat to people living with HIV, along with their sources of origin. Chapter 6, "Safe Food-Handling Practices," is dedicated to specific measures you can take to reduce possible exposure to these pathogens.

Pathogen	Sources of Contamination
Clostridium botulinum	Improperly sealed canned goods, cross-contamination
Campylobacter	Poultry, untreated water, undercooked meats
Clostridium perfringens	Foods held and served at room temperature

(also called "cafeteria germ")	for long periods of time, unwashed vegetables, cross-contamination
Cryptosporidium	Water, fecal matter, cross-contamination
E. coli	Undercooked beef, fecal matter, cross-contamination
Giardia	Water, fecal matter, cross-contamination
Listeria	Unpasteurized dairy products, fecal matter, cross-contamination
Staphylococcus aureus	Foods left at room temperature for long periods, cross-contamination
Salmonella	Undercooked poultry, eggs, cross-contamination

Though some varieties of food poisoning have their own characteristics, most share the same mild to severe flulike symptoms, which may indicate any number of other health problems. For this reason food poisoning can be very difficult for a doctor to diagnose quickly or accurately. It is important to work closely with your physician at the onset of any severe conditions, or if you have symptoms of a milder nature that linger more than three days.

Pathogen	Symptoms of Infection
Clostridium botulinum	Difficulty breathing and swallowing, double vision, droopy eyelids
Campylobacter	Muscle pain, headache, diarrhea, nausea
Clostridiun perfringens	Diarrhea, gas pains
Cryptosporidium	Profuse watery diarrhea, abdominal cramps, fever
E. coli	Severe abdominal cramps, watery diarrhea
Giardia	Diarrhea, vomiting, nausea, fever
Listeria	Sudden fever, chills, headache, diarrhea
Staphylococcus aureus	Diarrhea, vomiting, nausea, fever
Salmonella	Headache, abdominal pain, diarrhea, vomiting, nausea, fever

CHEMICAL PRESERVATIVES

Food preservatives have, no doubt, been used by manufacturers with a free hand, often indiscriminately. However, these chemicals are not simply the villains of marketing strategies; they fill the very real role of preventing food spoilage. Whatever the concerns may be about the long-range health effects of preservatives in foods (and this issue should be regarded with the utmost seriousness), the fact remains that before their advent, vastly greater numbers of people than now sickened and died every year due to food poisoning, to say nothing of the nutritional requirements that often went unmet due to the absence of produce and fresh meats. In a perfect world we would all have access to an abundance of the freshest raw ingredients, safely handled. Failing that, judicious use of preservatives assures us of safer food in continuing supply.

Safe Food-Handling Practices

CROSS-CONTAMINATION

We live in a country with one of the highest standards of sanitary practices in the world, with adequate and abundant refrigeration, and with streamlined shipping of perishable goods. However, food poisoning is still a common occurrence—primarily due to the manner in which food is handled in our kitchens. Improper food handling causes cross-contamination. Food poisoning from outright food spoilage is rare.

Cross-contamination is the unknowing transfer of a pathogen from one surface or substance, where its presence might be expected, to another surface or substance that would otherwise rightly be expected to be wholesome. To thoroughly understand how to prevent cross-contamination, it is necessary to examine the modes and habits that foster its occurrence.

At one stage or another many of the foods we eat are abundant with naturally occurring pathogens; it is one of the primary reasons that we cook our foods. For example, we know not to eat some foods raw, such as poultry or pork, because these foods may carry salmonella or trichinosis. But many people do not realize that the salmonella that might be present in raw chicken can find its way into our systems by routes other than the chicken it-self. Salmonella is a bacterium that can live on a dry, room-temperature surface for up to two months. It would therefore be possible to use a cutting board for raw chicken, clean it inade-quately afterward, and, fully two months later, cut up an apple (not normally a vehicle for salmonella), and contaminate it. The of-fending bacteria in such a case would be transferred from the chicken to the body via the cutting board via the apple. The orig-inal chicken? It was thoroughly cooked and caused no problems when eaten. Cross-contamination.

By far the most common vector for food poisoning in this coun-try is the humble can opener. Often used and seldom washed, it re-tains minute encrustations of food left on the blade to rot, providing a perfect culture for bacteria that are then forced into the contents of the next can opened. Frequently, canned goods are merely heated instead of being thoroughly cooked, thereby pro-ducing an ideal environment for the rapid multiplication of the of-fending bacteria.

Without question a can opener should be as thoroughly washed as any other kitchen utensil. In the case of electric can openers this is virtually impossible. For this reason they should be dis-carded. (Please note that you will be doing no one a favor by giv-ing it away.) Some brands of can openers state on their packaging labels that it is not necessary to wash them. Disregard that notice. It is presumably thought that the danger of the blade rusting slightly if washed outweighs in importance the possibility of gut-wrenching illness or death. While it is perfectly true that the blade will not remain sharp as long if frequently washed (drying the blade after rinsing will help minimize rust), the only possibly safe way to use can openers is to wash them thoroughly and replace them as often as necessary.

Other habits of kitchen routine will reveal many opportunities for cross-contamination. Let's examine some of the most common and the best means to avoid them.

Of course, washing is the first line of defense for the prevention of cross-contamination, and that which passes from every sub-stance we eat to every utensil we use or surface we work upon is our hands. That we should wash them thoroughly and frequently in hot soapy water, and always after handling something known to potentially harbor pathogens, such as poultry, should go without saying. Your mother and all of those grade-school teachers were right about this, as far as they went. They went, however, possibly not far enough. For example, with which hands did you turn on the faucet—those dripping with liquid from the raw chicken you've just put into a roasting pan? And after carefully washing, did you use those same handles to turn off the water? Cross-contamination. Did you lift the lid to the garbage can to throw away the packaging with those same wet hands, hours later to open it again to throw away a scrap of paper and afterward possibly touch your mouth? Again, cross-contamination. As you begin to examine your routines thoughtfully, you will no doubt recognize many instances in which cross-contamination is likely.

The point here is not to develop a hand-washing fetish, but to understand and avoid the actions that would foster the transfers. For instance, when your hands are not clean, you may find that you can open the garbage-can lid with your foot or the dry back of your hand. A faucet handle might be nudged on with an elbow. One quickly becomes a contortionist realizing the paths of conta-mination and circumventing them. Or you might leave a dish rag in the sink for the very purpose of using it to grasp the faucet han-dles, washing it out as you wash your hands. The use of paper towels instead of cloth towels will also help reduce the chance of cross-contamination. **Note that antibacterial soaps are not de-signed to sanitize, but merely to reduce surface bacteria of a sort that causes body odor; they are not effective against food-poisoning bacteria. The thoroughness of the washing is your safeguard here.**

Raw foodstuffs are handled not only in the kitchen, but also in the market while shopping. Raw meats, poultry, and fish provide the greatest threats to safety for the dual reasons that, first, they are naturally abundant sources of pathogens and, second, their packaging frequently leaks. Blood or other liquids, even by droplets, can contaminate a whole shopping cart full of food, or your hands when handling the wet packages. From there you may contaminate the steering wheel of your car, the handle of your refrigerator as you put away groceries, the milk or other containers as you put them away, and so on. Better to contain such packages safely in the first place.

The easiest way to contain the packages is to use the plastic bags available in many meat and almost all produce sections **even as you pick up packages to look at them.** Simply slip your hand inside a bag as though it were an oversized mitten. When you have found the package you desire, just turn the bag "inside out" over the package while still holding it with your "mittened" hand. You will have contained the package without ever touching it. A twist closed, and this will not only serve as an (almost) leakproof way to bring foods home, but also to store them in the refrigerator.

Another course of cross-contamination is to use the same utensils from the beginning to the end of the cooking process without washing them. Summer grilling is an excellent example, where many people place raw meat on a grill, turn the half-cooked meat, and remove the cooked meat with the same fork. They then replace the meat on the same platter they carried it out on and which has sat in the summer heat throughout the cooking, neither fork nor platter having been washed in the interval. This, of course, applies not only to grilling practices, but to any multiple-step cooking processes throughout which we repeatedly handle foods.

SAFE FOOD SELECTION

Food safety also requires prudent marketing strategies. Pick up nonperishable foods (such as canned, dried, or bottled goods) before perishables, so that the perishables are out of refrigeration as short a time as possible. Make the food market the last stop on your excursion and go straight home after shopping for groceries. A car's air conditioner does not supply sufficient cooling to keep cold foods cold. In hot weather, consider carrying a cooler to transport refrigerated perishables, especially if you must be outside for any length of time. Remember to keep that cooler clean. Put perishables away as soon as you get home.

Don't buy canned goods with dents, rust, or bulges, even if they are on sale. Do not buy foods past their freshness date. These dates are general guidelines only, reflecting optimal handling conditions. Many occurrences, including casual handling by market employees and customers, can compromise the freshness of an individual package. Only use pasteurized milk products. This excludes many aged or ripened cheeses.

In general, pay attention to the level of cleanliness in a market, including that of the food handlers themselves. Though this is an uncertain index at best, be assured that if you can see unsanitary practices, things are worse where you cannot see. Most frequently, lack of sanitation is inadvertent or uninformed, but all of the dangers of cross-contamination still exist, intentional or no. Cooked shrimps, for example, displayed on a bed of crushed ice next to raw seafood is a common breach of safe food-handling practices and reflects a lack of awareness on the part of the staff and management. Shop in delicatessens and salad bars only at your own risk. Unlike other perishables (such as dairy products, which are sealed, or meats, which are to be cooked), it is impossible to know the freshness and wholesomeness of these foods, which are most often eaten as purchased. If food-handling practices here should be below par, cross-contamination may have occurred. Caveat emptor. (Buyer beware!)

SANITIZING WORK SURFACES

Soap and hot water are our best allies. There is nothing that replaces the thorough washing of surfaces, hands, and utensils to reduce the presence of naturally occurring pathogens. However, to really sanitize surfaces, cooks at home would be wise to follow the same guidelines established by health departments for food-service industries. After washing, use a mild solution of chlorinated water to sterilize countertops, cutting boards, and periodically the refrigerator. That pesky can opener, too, can be dunked in the solution after being washed, to assure cleanliness in all of its little nooks and crannies. The recommended proportions are as follows:

1 quart water
1 tablespoon liquid chlorine bleach (such as Clorox)

This simple solution will sanitize more effectively than a host of fancy commercial cleaners, and should have a designated place in a working kitchen. Some health-department regulations require that a bucket of bleach water be on each and every work space in a professional kitchen. Please note that the solution mixed in the proportion above is quite adequate to sanitize surfaces; increasing the amount of chlorine will only cause pitting and corrosion of surfaces, but no additional sterilization.

As chlorine is volatile, it is necessary to make the solution fresh every day you work in the kitchen. For those concerned about exposure to chlorine, be assured that: 1) chlorine dissipates rapidly and harmlessly into the air as it is swabbed over surfaces, and 2) the slight exposure to chlorine used this way is a fraction of that to which we are exposed every day in our drinking and bath waters. Anyone who has swum in a pool has been exposed to much greater quantities. Short of drinking this solution, it will do you no harm. **WARNING: CHLORINE BLEACH SHOULD NOT BE COMBINED WITH ANY OTHER CLEANERS OR CHEMICAL SOLUTIONS, AS THE COMBINATION POTENTIALLY CAN PRODUCE EXTREMELY HARMFUL GASES.** Such cleaners include ammonia, dishwashing liquids, floor cleaners, and scouring powders, among others.

The easiest way to incorporate sanitizing with chlorinated water into your kitchen routine is to choose a bowl that will hold over a quart of liquid and designate it solely for that purpose. Pour in a measured quart of water and see where it comes to in the bowl.

Mark a line, if you like, or fix the spot in your memory, so that in the future you can measure your water "by eye" at the tap. Find a tablespoon measure to use as a bleach measure, and reserve it, too, so that it is handy and you can measure easily. A flip-top squeeze bottle will make pouring and measuring bleach more convenient and accurate. The idea is to make this as effortless and routine as possible. It should become as habitual as washing your hands or returning perishables to the refrigerator.

Be advised that bleach in the kitchen acts just as it does in the laundry, and if bleach is splashed it will leave spots, especially on dark clothing. For that reason you may wish to reserve some old clothes for working in the kitchen, or choose a time-honored solution: wear an apron. Sponges, too, will disintegrate faster than one would think possible if allowed to remain in the bleach water. Therefore, only saturate them when they're being used, and rinse them afterward. Dishrags may be preferable, as they tend to hold up better for this purpose.

The question is frequently asked whether the bleach solution can be used in an atomizer, and kept for several days, since it is a closed container from which the chlorine will not dissipate. Generally speaking, no, but the answer really depends on how you use the atomizer. For the bleach solution to sterilize, surfaces must be thoroughly wetted with it. Without a great deal of effort atomizers usually produce only a light mist, which is not only insufficient to sanitize, but also hard to control in its application. For these reasons atomizers are not suggested.

Sanitizing with chlorinated water is an adjunct, not an alternative, to thorough washing and cannot be solely relied upon to make safe otherwise unclean surfaces.

REFRIGERATION

For refrigeration to have its optimal effect of keeping food fresh and safe, the temperature needs to be kept within a certain range. In the freezer that means below 0 degrees Fahrenheit (minus 18 degrees Celsius); in the refrigerator, between 34 and 40 degrees

THE GREAT CUTTING-BOARD DEBATE

There has been much press given in the last several years to a research project at the University of Wisconsin, which concluded (contrary to conventional wisdom and popular expectations) that wooden cutting boards are safer than those made of plastic, due to the natural antibacterial qualities of the wood's resins. Studies at the National Sanitation Foundation and at the Food and Drug Administration have not been able to replicate these findings. Their studies indicate that there is no regular quantitative difference in growth-support potential on either substance, plastic or wood. While the actual substance of the cutting boards may be equal, their structure and the mechanics of their use are very different in their ability to harbor bacteria. The porous nature of wood makes it impossible to clean thoroughly. This problem is exacerbated by the common alternate use of wooden cutting boards as hot plates, which encourages bacteria to grow deep into the wood's fibers, where it is protected. Later, when cutting against and into the wood, those bacteria are exposed, and cross-contamination can occur. Plastic, which is impervious, can be cleaned and sanitized much more thoroughly.

For greatest safety it is best to have two cutting boards: one reserved for raw meats, fish, and poultry and the other set aside for cooked foods and those foods, such as fruits and vegetables, that are eaten raw. In this way the danger of cross-contamination via cutting boards is reduced to an absolute minimum.

Fahrenheit (1 to 5 degrees Celsius). Many refrigerators fail in this, due to overcrowding or frost buildup. Sometimes their thermostats are simply not set low enough. As it is impossible to gauge the chill of a refrigerator accurately in any other way, a refrigerator thermometer is advisable to monitor temperature. Though most bacteria multiply at an increasingly faster rate as the temperature warms to room temperature, the 40-degree mark is something of a dividing line, above which the acceleration rate is most dramatic. For purposes of freezing the dividing line is 0 degrees.

Freezing, still less refrigeration, does not destroy food-poisoning pathogens but merely arrests their development. While it is all too clear that things can spoil in the refrigerator (how's that "science project" doing?), spoilage can also occur in the freezer if the bulk of warm food is too great and the chill of the freezer insufficient to rapidly freeze the food. This is to say nothing of freezer burn from extended storage, which, though harmless, can render foods tough and tasteless. It is wise to store foods wrapped carefully, dated, and not longer than the recommendations below:

Fruits and Vegetables	**1 year or less**
Red Meat	**9 months or less**
Poultry	**6 months or less**
Ground Meats	**3 months or less**
Fish—fat (salmon, trout, mackerel)	**3 months or less**
—lean (flounder, snapper, haddock)	**6 months or less**

Improper thawing of frozen foods is another potentially dangerous area for the rapid multiplication of bacteria. For example: The surface half inch of a frozen turkey left on a kitchen counter can thaw to room temperature while the core is still frozen rock solid. In that half inch rampant bacterial activity can occur. It is therefore important to thaw frozen foods in the refrigerator, where the entire item is assured of continued chill while the thawing takes place. Of course, this takes much longer, so some advanced planning is necessary. Thinner, smaller packages will thaw at a faster rate than those of greater bulk. Very generally, in properly cold refrigeration, a large roast or turkey will take four to seven hours **per pound** to thaw, while a small roast or bird will take only three to five hours per pound. When thawing foods in the refrigerator, as when storing raw food, it is important not to let them leak onto other foods. Even something that seemed to have no fluid when it went into the freezer can drip as it thaws, due to the cell-membrane disruption caused by freezing. Place any thawing food into a pan or bowl, so that it won't drip onto and contaminate other foods.

If it is necessary to thaw something more rapidly, doing so either in a microwave oven or in a basin of cool running water is recommended. For this latter, have the frozen object in a leak-proof plastic bag and place it in a bowl larger than itself. Put the bowl in a sink and let *cold* water run over it, overflowing the bowl and draining into the sink. Do not rush this process by using hot or warm water, or you can foster the same surface spoilage problem described above. Let the water continue to run slowly and check the package frequently. If it is something that may be broken apart upon partial thawing, such as cut-up chicken, loosen it as soon as conveniently possible and return it to the cold running water until just thawed. Promptly cook all foods upon thawing.

Foods that have been thoroughly cooked are sterile, since the heating process destroys the native bacteria residing in it. However, airborne pathogens will quickly reestablish colonies of bacterial growth in foods if they are left out at room temperature for long. To retard this process it is therefore necessary to refrigerate hot foods as soon as possible. A word of caution here: Most home refrigerators do not have sufficiently rapid recovery of cooling to prevent the entire contents of a refrigerator from warming to well above 40 degrees if either a large quantity of warm food or something really blazing hot is put into it. Therefore monitor hot foods until they have cooled to lukewarm and then promptly put them away. Foods stored in several small containers will cool more quickly than a single large package. Leaving lids ajar until the cooling is complete will help heat to escape, but all stored foods should be carefully covered afterward, using sealable containers, plastic wrap, or aluminum foil.

Eggs should be left stored in their cartons in the refrigerator for two reasons. First, eggs are packed in their cartons blunt end up, which is the optimal position for their safe storage. Secondly, as most egg storage compartments are in the doors of refrigerators, eggs there are exposed to blasts of warm air every time the door is opened. The carton provides a degree of insulation that helps maintain a constant chill. Eggs should always be kept under refrigeration, as every day at room temperature causes nutritional loss equal to that of a week in the refrigerator. It is *not* necessary to wash eggs: in fact, there is a natural antibacterial coating to the egg that is water soluble and whose protective properties would thus be lost. If you feel that you must do so, wash them only just before using. Finally, never use a cracked egg; the financial expense is too slight and the potential cost to your health is too great.

There is no hard-and-fast rule as to the length of time food may be safely stored in the refrigerator. Too many variables influence the keeping properties of any single food, much less a multiplicity of foods. Therefore, the bottom-line golden rule is always: **When in doubt, throw it out! Without tasting it!** Generally, leftovers kept more than two or three days are questionable unless they are subjected to a *thorough* recooking and not merely reheating (e.g., leftover turkey baked in a casserole). Better to cook in smaller quantities or to freeze leftovers promptly than to continue to eat food whose safety has become suspect. Much.

Safe Cooking Guidelines

Thorough cooking will destroy virtually all natural pathogens. If food should be contaminated with chemical toxins such as cleaning solution, it cannot be made safe to eat and should be scrupulously avoided.

It is one of the great culinary losses that commonly, in an attempt to assure safety, many foods are cooked far beyond the point necessary to render them safe. The accurate gauging of internal temperatures is impossible for even the most experienced of cooks without using a thermometer. The only way to know accurately the temperature of food as it cooks is to use an instant reading thermometer. This item can be used to monitor not only roasts and casseroles, but anything else you may cook, including liquids such as soups and stews. You may even use this same thermometer to gauge the temperature of your refrigerator.

An instant reading thermometer is different from the old fashioned "meat thermometer," which is an inaccurate gauge at best. The latter is left in a roast as it cooks, conducting heat along its metal shaft, so that what it actually measures is not the internal temperature of the roast, but that of a narrow sleeve of meat along the shaft, which cooks faster due to the localized heat transfer.

The shaft of a meat thermometer is approximately the diameter of a ballpoint pen, and its dial, usually square, two to three inches across.

By contrast, an instant reading thermometer has a much narrower shaft and a round dial slightly less than that of a quarter in diameter. It is used by plunging it into the thickest part of whatever is being cooked until it hits the pan or a bone, and then retracting it slightly. After several seconds the dial should register an accurate reading. DO NOT LEAVE IT IN THE DISH IN THE OVEN, EVEN FOR A FEW MINUTES, OR IT WILL BE RUINED! To measure the temperature of a liquid, simply place the shaft into the liquid without touching the pan. *Tip:* If steam from a hot liquid makes this difficult, the thermometer may be suspended through the tines of a fork. You may also test your thermometer's accuracy by trying this with boiling water. Water boils at 212 degrees Fahrenheit: if your thermometer registers other than 212, either return it to the store for a replacement or always remember to add or subtract the variation from any subsequent readings, as the relative scale should remain constant. In measuring roasts or other dishes of large, solid bulk, be aware that the internal temperature will continue to rise between 5 and 10 degrees after it has been taken from the oven. It is therefore necessary to remove such things slightly before the target temperature is reached in order to avoid overcooking.

Inexplicably, the cost of these very standard items varies wildly, commonly ranging from $2.95 in restaurant supply stores to $12.95 in fancy kitchenware shops. THERE IS NO QUALITATIVE DIFFERENCE. Buy the cheap one.

Assuming, then, the ability to measure the temperature of foods accurately, let's look at the internal temperature necessary to assure safety.

---

160 degrees

To many, that number will come as a surprise, if not a shock. Many older guides recommend minimum internal temperatures up to 190 degrees. More good food has been ruined by unnecessary overcooking in the name of safety than for just about any other reason. Two hundred years ago the art of cooking was mainly the art of spicing. For lack of refrigeration and preservatives most foods were simply stewed to oblivion in order to assure their safety. Old customs die hard, and we still live with the legacy and notions of those times. It is hardly any wonder that people lose their interest in food when they are told everything must be cooked well done, the general assumption being that this means cooked to death. Well done (indicating thoroughly cooked) means 160 degrees or above.

You may find that you prefer many foods even further cooked for reasons of taste. Poultry cooked to 160 degrees, while safe, seems rather raw to most tastes. Pork, from time immemorial, has been cooked to a far greater degree of doneness than 160 degrees, and so history shaped our tastes of what cooked pork is supposed to be. You may find that pork cooked to an internal temperature of 160 degrees seems raw and unappealing. You may, on the other hand, find it succulent and ambrosial. The point here is not to talk anyone into eating meats too rare for his taste, but rather to assure those who prefer rarer meats that they need not cook them to such a degree of doneness as to destroy their appeal, in the erroneous and misguided notion that food safety requires it.

One hundred sixty degrees is the minimum safe internal temperature for meat and poultry as established by the U.S. Department of Agriculture, Food Safety, and Inspection Service. Cooking beyond this point does not produce any greater degree of sterilization. However, **when in doubt,** erring on the side of caution assures safety. For example, when you are eating away from home and cannot accurately gauge the internal temperature of a meat (a steak ordered in a restaurant, for example), it is always safest to select a degree of doneness that will assure this minimum. When at home, by cooking foods to a **slightly** higher internal temperature than 160 degrees you will assure that no recessed pockets, shielded perhaps by bone or connective tissue, have failed to reach the adequate minimum.

For some foods there are simply not convenient methods to measure their temperatures (scrambled eggs, for example), and we must rely on other indicators to determine if cooking has been sufficient and complete. Traditional tests generally indicate a degree of doneness beyond what is minimally necessary, but it is frequently only in those states of doneness that conclusive visual cues exist.

EGGS

Fresh eggs, a possible and ready source of salmonella, should be cooked until firm. This means no "sunny side up," "over easy," soft scrambled, or soft boiled eggs. No lightly cooked custards or sauces, such as hollandaise or béarnaise, and nothing uncooked made from fresh eggs, such as eggnog. This last category is larger than perhaps it seems at first glance. No tasting raw batters or cookie doughs. In addition, Caesar and other salad dressings are typically made with raw egg, as is homemade mayonnaise, and all should be avoided. Please note that commercially produced mayonnaise has been pasteurized and presents no undue risk. In fact, with its mild acid content it is actually slightly resistant to spoilage. The myth of mayonnaise being particularly susceptible to bacterial action and therefore a looming danger in all of that picnic-bound potato salad is just that: a myth. Any of the above-mentioned foods may be prepared safely using pasteurized eggs. These are available frozen in several different brands (such as Egg Beaters).

MEATS

While larger cuts of meats are ideally tested for doneness using an instant reading thermometer, it is simply not feasible with many smaller cuts, such as chicken legs. For these pieces, whether meat or poultry, the standard test is that the juices should run clear when the meat is pierced with a fork. Red meat should be just beyond pink to gray. Again, please do not think that this means food must be cooked until it is tough and dry—"Reduced to cinders," as the French say. Doing so will only lessen your pleasure without adding any measure of safety. It should be noted that the dark red streaks one occasionally encounters near the bone in poultry are not blood or evidence of insufficient cooking, but rather immature marrow that has leaked out of the bone during cooking. It is quite harmless.

GROUND MEATS

Ground meats, including hamburger, sausages, and turkey, present extra risk beyond that of meat in general for three important reasons: 1) Ground meat is handled more than any other raw meat product. 2) With its vast and vulnerable surface area due to grinding, potential exposure to pathogens is much greater. 3) The cleanliness of massive meat grinders, with all of their nooks and crannies, may be less than desired.

Perhaps the greatest potential danger from ground meat comes from hamburger in large-scale manufacture. In mass-produced hamburger it is possible that a single pattie can contain bits and traces of up to two hundred cows (a staggering thought) and if any one of them is infected with any pathogen, all of the meat is thereby contaminated. If your immune system is very fragile, but you are devoted to hamburger, small quantities of meat may be ground in a food processor or an old-fashioned meat grinder (these can usually be found quite cheap at yard sales and the like). Grinding your own meat, where you can know the quality and wholesomeness of the meat and determine for yourself the necessary sanitation practices, is not difficult and is your greatest assurance of safety. This is not to suggest that all ground meats are unsafe; merely that safe handling and thorough cooking are of particular concern.

PORK

Pork is one of the foods most commonly destroyed by unnecessary overcooking due to well-known concerns about the threat of trichinosis. The fact is that trichinosis is *extremely* rare in this country, occurring when it does virtually always from under-cooked wild game. Hogs in commercial production are individually tested for the parasite, and meat from those in which it is discovered (less than 1 percent) is routed for processed-food production, which assures its sterilization. The 160-degree rule applies to pork as to other meats, and you may be surprised to notice that at that internal temperature there is often still a slight trace of pink showing. The old rule requiring pork cooked until no pink shows existed to visually indicate the point at which it was certain that pork was on the far side of doneness.

FISH AND SEAFOOD

No fish or seafood should ever be eaten raw. This includes raw clams and oysters, sushi, and seviche. It is a matter of lively debate as to whether anyone in the general population should be eating this, but if you are immunocompromised, doing so is really asking for trouble. All fish should be cooked until it flakes when prodded with a fork. It should be opaque, with no translucence or rubberiness remaining. Shellfish, if steamed, should be cooked until thoroughly done.

STUFFING

Cooking poultry with stuffing is a potentially risky undertaking for several reasons. The stuffing is exposed to the raw bird (and therefore possibly toxic bacteria) as it is placed inside. Buried deeply, it may never be cooked sufficiently to destroy such bacteria. Rather, it may instead be heated to a temperature at which the bacteria will proliferate. In fact, roasting a bird long enough to heat a stuffing to the point of safety frequently means the fowl will be overcooked. Starchy bread or rice stuffings provide ideal settings in which the bacteria may grow well, and if the stuffing is not removed from the bird soon after cooking, the chance is that it will remain for so long in the "danger zone" of temperature, that, even if it is refrigerated, spoilage may occur. You may test stuffing in several places with your instant reading thermometer and if it consistently reaches 160 degrees or above, it is sufficiently cooked. Still, it is far safer to serve "dressing" that has been baked simultaneously outside the bird. Make it with broth and baste it with drippings while cooking to replicate the flavor of stuffing.

PARTIAL OR INTERRUPTED COOKING

If the final cooking of food brings its internal temperature to 160 degrees or above, the food will have been rendered sterile. However, partial cooking reaching below this temperature is apt only to provide an environment in which bacteria multiply prolifically. Should the subsequent cooking prove insufficient, the vastly more abundant pathogen will provide a much greater threat than would normally be encountered. Therefore, all cooking should be done in a single, complete operation.

SLOW COOKERS

Also called Crock-Pot cookers, these are excellent, safe ways to cook, as they reach and maintain a temperature above the minimum 160 degrees needed to assure safety. (For more about slow cookers, see page 150.)

MICROWAVE COOKING

Microwave cooking is a convenient adjunct to many kitchen routines. Despite the dire warnings of many detractors, microwave cooking has now been around for half a century and is perfectly safe as long as certain guidelines are followed. Failing those, it can become a potent vector of unsafely cooked food and therefore of food poisoning.

As anyone who has experience with a microwave oven lacking a turntable knows, the heating can be extremely localized. A small slice of frozen cheesecake, for example, can be reduced to molten slag on one end while retaining frost crystals on the other. No type of microwave oven has completely surmounted this problem, though those with turntables (which may be bought separately) are much more efficient at even, thorough cooking. Because of this localized heating phenomenon, the *technique* of cooking in a microwave is necessarily different. Those intermittent and post-cooking "rest" times in recipes and heating instructions for convenience foods are not merely designed to frustrate the impatient diner, but rather to allow heat transfer to equalize throughout the food being cooked. To neglect these waiting periods causes the very likely risk that uncooked areas will remain in the food.

To cook safely using a microwave oven, it is best not to cook meats containing bones, as bones can shield the surrounding meat from microwave bombardment and thereby exacerbate the problem of localized heating. Keeping food in regularly shaped pieces and in evenly distributed, shallow layers in the cooking container will also help standardize cooking. Covering foods with plastic wrap is suggested to facilitate heat diffusion. Cooking at medium power, which is slower, will help too. The internal temperature of food cooked in a microwave can, of course, be verified using an instant reading thermometer. Manufacturers' instructions for individual packaged items have been carefully worked out and their guidelines should be followed.

Another important reason to observe the post-cooking rest times has to do with the very manner in which microwave ovens generate heat. Heat is produced by extra-short radio waves which cause molecular agitation. As the molecules rub together, their friction creates heat. Molecular agitation can continue in food even after the food is no longer being bombarded by the radio waves—up to ten minutes in the instance of some foods with long cooking times. This means that if something is eaten directly from microwave cooking, unlike other hot foods which may be gauged as to their heat as we eat them, MICROWAVED FOOD CAN CONTINUE TO **GENERATE** HEAT EVEN IN THE STOMACH! Resting guidelines in microwave-cooking instructions should be scrupulously observed.

8

Water Safety

Concern over the safety of the nation's water supply is growing as infrastructures decay, consciousness is raised, and incidents of cryptosporidium and giardia,* waterborne parasites resistant to most common forms of purification treatments, continue to spread. While the great majority of water sources are safe most of the time, flooding or other temporary conditions can sometimes pollute any given water supply. The effect of contamination can be both great and unremitting on someone whose immune system is compromised—devastating, in fact, for those whose immune systems are very fragile.

Doubtless some of you reading this are supplied water by your municipality, others have your own private wells. Because water sources are so varied and since scrutiny has only recently begun prompting improvement of testing and treatment in many water departments throughout the country, it is impossible to give a list which is both current and exhaustive of the water supplies that are

---

* Cryptosporidium and giardia, one-celled organisms that thrive in the intestinal tracts of mammals, are the most common and virulent infectious agents found in water supplies, though others, such as salmonella, can also be waterborne.

secure. The following guidelines will allow you to determine whether your own water source is safe and, if not, what steps you might take to see that its safety is restored.

Contamination occurs largely in surface water, as opposed to deep spring or artesian well water which comes from the aquifer. Surface water includes the lakes, streams, and reservoirs that supply most of our water and also water from regular (not artesian) wells. Although chemical contamination is certainly possible, it is quite rare in the protected water reserves that supply our municipalities or in modern wells that have been properly situated and drilled. The far greater risk of contamination is of animal origin. Pasture runoff, for example, can transfer oocysts (the egg stage of parasites such as cryptosporidium) from fecal matter to ground water.* Not only are these oocysts so extremely small that they are able to pass through most filtration systems (a million can fit in an eight-ounce glass of water), but they are also impervious to chlorination, which is the standard method of water treatment. Some authorities estimate that 85 percent of all surface water in this country is infected with cryptosporidium; for this reason no untreated water should be considered potable. Though the water that forms our water reservoirs is somewhat protected, it is not inviolable. Further, occasional flooding may cause sewer backups to leak into water systems, causing localized and temporary contamination.

What to do? This is not an easy question. The answer depends in part on how vulnerable your own immune system is and the degree of effort you're willing to put into prevention efforts.

First, you may contact your local water department to determine what precautions, if any, they take to prevent such contamination. Be forewarned that water departments have a vested interest in assuring the public that water supplies are safe. Evasive language (doublespeak) is frequently raised to an art form in this, as in other,

---

* Because these organisms are fecally transferred, scrupulous hygiene (i.e., thorough hand washing) must be maintained with respect to toilet use by all those who share an environment with someone living with AIDS. In addition, any sexual activity that includes oral/anal or fecal contact should be avoided entirely.

bureaucracies. Ask to speak to an engineer and discuss with him/her what monitoring, testing, or treatment is done to address this problem and what, if any, known incidents have occurred in the last several years. As these diseases have been recognized relatively recently (since the mid-1970s), and as proper testing, much less treatment, of water is elaborate and expensive, many water departments will have no safeguards in place. The Environmental Protection Agency operates a Safe Drinking Water Hotline ([800] 426-4791), which should be able to give you some information about your local municipal water supply. Alternately, you may check with your local AIDS service organization to see if they have made or will make these inquiries. If your water supply is a private well, contact your local agricultural extension agent or county health department to learn what testing is available in your area.

Most water supplies are safe most of the time. If you feel you have reason to suspect the safety of your water (such as incidents of cryptosporidium in your community) you have several options.

BOILING WATER

One option is to boil your water. Any water not chemically contaminated can be rendered safe and sterile by bringing it to a rolling boil for one full minute. Kept in the covered container in which it was boiled (which will have been sterilized by the process), it will remain safe indefinitely as long as it is not contaminated by the introduction of pathogens through being left uncovered or by contact with unclean hands or utensils. It may also be transferred to a clean, *dry* container, preferably covered. Please note that this transfer is most safely made after the water has had a chance to cool.

As it can take quite a while to bring any large quantity of water to a boil, always begin with the hottest tap water available and keep the container covered with a close-fitting lid. If you decide to make this a regular practice, you may find a large stockpot helpful. Some are made with a spigot near the bottom, which makes it possible to draw water without removing the lid.

BOTTLED WATERS

Another option is to use bottled water. Do *not,* however, assume the mere fact of a water's having been bottled as a guarantee of safety in these matters. Some waters are bottled from the bottler's municipal water with no further treatment of any kind (meaning straight from the tap). Others are treated by methods not adequate to address this problem.

All distilled water is considered safe and sterile. For any other water, surface or spring, filtration down to a minute degree (*absolute* one micron or less—"nominal" one micron is not sufficient) assures safety. Water treated by reverse osmosis is also safe. Springwater, being a "deep-source" versus "surface" water, is very unlikely to be contaminated by cryptosporidiosis. In fact, the International Bottled Water Association considers any bottled springwater safe from cryptosporidium merely by virtue of its being springwater. This does NOT, however, meet the Centers for Disease Control's guidelines for absolute assurance. Do not be misled by the meaningless terms *spring-like* or *spring-type* seen occasionally on labels. The following is a partial list of bottlers whose waters comply with standards of filtration sufficient to prevent the presence of cryptosporidium.

BOTTLED WATERS PROCESSED TO ASSURE SAFETY FROM
CRYPTOSPORIDIUM*

Deer Park	Saratoga
Great Bear	Vivanti
Naya	Wissahickon
Poland Springs	

* You may note that Évian, one of the most famous bottled waters in the world, does not appear on the list. Although Évian comes from a deep-source aquifer and is therefore unlikely to be contaminated with cryptosporidium, no filtration or processing is performed that would guarantee its absence, nor is it tested specifically for cryptosporidium. This is another example of how price and reputation are not necessarily an assurance of sanitation.

Doubtless many other regional bottled waters meet the requirements necessary to safeguard against cryptosporidium. To determine this, call the customer-service representative of the bottler in question and ask if their water is either filtered to one micron or has been treated by reverse osmosis.

Some companies whose product meets these requirements supply home delivery of bottled waters, a great advantage if it is available, since hauling water can become exhausting. An added consideration is that you must maintain the cleanliness of the dispensing unit that holds the inverted bottle of water. Any moist dark place, over time, can breed bacteria and algae. To prevent this, mildly chlorinated water (one tablespoon chlorine bleach to one quart of the sterile water) should be flushed through the system once a month, followed by fresh water.

WATER FILTERS

Another alternative to ensure water safety is to install a water filtration system that will filter to one micron or less. This degree of filtration is NOT accomplished by casual countertop units such as the Brita system or most "on-the-tap" filters such as the Instapure Water Pik water filters. Only Class #1 filtration systems with a National Sanitation Foundation certification "NSF Standard 53 Cyst Removal" are adequate. These systems typically require installation under the counter, which a plumber or average do-it-yourselfer can easily accomplish. A number of companies (such as Everpure) produce filtration systems to this standard, designed for a variety of commercial and domestic applications (such as for travel). Recently the PUR company has produced an on-the-tap filter with a Standard 53 rating that retails for about fifty dollars. For a complete and current free list of manufacturers of water filtration systems approved by the National Sanitation Foundation, along with makes, models, and ratings, call (800) 673-8010. Larger-capacity under-the-counter systems typically begin at a little under two hundred dollars and move upward. In the long run either type supplies safe water much more cheaply than purchased bottled water (approximately seven to eighteen cents a gallon) and if used correctly are very efficient. All systems require periodic replacement of their filters (frequency depending upon usage), and customer noncompliance in prompt filter replacement is by far the most common cause of failure to provide safe water. The PUR filter has an automatic shutoff feature when the filter is used to capacity, additionally recommending it.

If you have concluded that your regular supply of water is not secure to prevent infection and have therefore decided to rely on boiled, bottled, or filtered water, it is necessary to practice this as a complete regimen. To drink a glass of bottled water and reconstitute your frozen orange juice with (contaminated) tap water would, of course, be pointless. The water you use when you are brushing your teeth, however, may be a less obvious but nonetheless real opportunity for infection. Since freezing does not destroy the parasites, ice is only as safe as the water it is made from, and this includes commercially produced ice. Numerous examples of infection exist from perfectly safe beverages cross-contaminated with ice produced in plants whose water supply was contaminated or whose facility sanitation was below par. Water is also ingested in foods such as soups. (Please note that often canned soups are reconstituted and if you only heat them to serving temperature it is inadequate heat to destroy cryptosporidium.) All of the water you are exposed to must therefore be safeguarded. When bathing, showering, or swimming, keep the water out of your mouth.

The question arises as to the possibility of cross-contamination from eating and cooking utensils washed and rinsed in tap water. These are considered safe if they have been allowed to dry *thoroughly,* preferably air (or dishwasher-cycle) dried, not towel dried. The reason for this is that the oocysts, while extremely hardy in many adversarial environments (such as chlorinated water) and able to live for long periods of time in moisture, are very vulnerable to desiccation (drying out) and are thus quickly destroyed.

As noted elsewhere, we live not in a vacuum but a real world, and in such there will always be threats, immunocompromised or not. Water is such an omnipresent part of our lives that it is impossible to safeguard ourselves in every particular at every moment. Having taken the precautions available to us and recognizing the compromises necessary, we need to continue the business of living our lives.

9

Eating Defensively Away from Home

The earlier chapters of this section outline the considerations necessary for the safe handling and cooking of foods. As long as we respect these guidelines, food safety and freedom from food poisoning are relatively easy to assure. But what do we do when we are away from home and cannot know or control the sanitary conditions? In this chapter we will deal with defensive eating practices that offer the greatest safety, though you should be advised that, especially through the risk of cross-contamination, virtually any food can be a potential source of food-borne illness.

Most of us have been told all of our lives that if we ever saw the inside of a restaurant kitchen, we would never eat in another restaurant as long as we lived. I have worked in a number of restaurants through the years and for the most part haven't found that to be true. *However,* if I may be permitted an anecdote: I once worked, briefly, in a restaurant of national reputation where the food-safety standards were staggeringly low. Untrained and unskilled kitchen workers would stand in the sweltering heat cutting up raw chicken on wooden cutting tables by the hour. If someone from the salad station would yell down that he needed more cucumber sliced quickly, the mound of warm, raw chicken would be pushed to the side of the table and, with no further preliminaries, cucumbers would be cut. From one day to the next these tables would be given only the barest wipe-down. This is but one example of the many breaches of safe food handling that occurred there daily. My complaints to those in charge fell on deaf ears; I could only see to it that my area of the kitchen and those who worked under me maintained sanitary practices. I did not stay there long. To this day you can buy this restaurant's cookbook in many bookstores throughout the country. Reputation does not assure sanitation.

What to do, then? First of all, assume the worst. Restaurants are low-profit-margin businesses whose economic viability frequently depends on low-paid workers who are consequently unskilled and generally uneducated. Lack of sanitation is due not so much to an evil plot as it is to apathy and a lack of knowledge. If those in charge are not personally committed to food safety, that attitude gets passed down the chain of command and is quickly lost in the toot and scramble of restaurant life. Therefore, size up the situation. If a place does not seem adequately clean—leave. It is not necessary to make any explanation. If you choose to do so (and it would serve the cause of food safety well if restaurant owners knew that they were losing business on the basis of this criterion), call the next day and speak to a manager. If you register a complaint at the time of departure, several things are likely: 1) If you do talk to the manager, she, in the heat of the mealtime rush, is likely not to pay much attention, whereas she might be much more receptive at a less busy time; 2) if you speak to a subordinate, the message is not apt to be delivered to anyone who might address the problem; 3) you might find yourself in an awkward and embarrassing situation as, defensively, someone tries to persuade you that you are wrong; and finally, 4) if the problem is of sufficient magnitude to have caused concern in the first place, it probably cannot be corrected before preparation for your meal begins—in some cases days before you got there. If you must offer some explanation to the people with whom you are dining, simply state the truth: "The place didn't seem clean."

How to gauge this? It is a haphazard area at best, but (and I say this on the basis of many years' restaurant experience), at the risk of sounding like one of those "dear old aunties," cleanliness of the rest rooms is as reliable an index as one may find. If the management is so completely uninterested in its public face of cleanliness, you may be assured that hygiene is not a particular concern of theirs. Things are undoubtedly worse where you cannot see. Perhaps you can "answer nature's call" even before being seated and, if necessary, upon your return announce quietly that you've changed your mind. No explanation needed. Beyond this you must use your critical and intuitive faculties to assess as best you may.

Assuming, then, that you have decided upon a restaurant, let's further consider how you may make intelligent choices to avoid the risk of food poisoning.

To start with, the reader ought to learn, at home, to recognize visually the degree of doneness of foods she might order later in the restaurant. Do this by using an instant reading thermometer as was described in Chapter 7, "Safe Cooking Guidelines." Having a visual reference will prove an invaluable guide to gauging the doneness of whatever is served you when eating out. Erring on the side of caution, it is safest to order meats "just on the far side of pink," as a minimum degree of doneness—or beyond that to whatever degree you prefer. Special concern should be given hamburger, as ground meats are the most susceptible to bacterial attack and therefore the most perishable. Think nothing of sending food back, however many times it may take, until it is at the degree of doneness you have specified. This includes meats that are too far cooked as well as those that are too rare. Using specific descriptive terms such as *pinkness* usually brings more accurate results than general terms, such as *medium well,* for which virtually every cook and diner has a different index.

Thoroughly cooked foods served hot are safest. For the reasons illustrated in the anecdote earlier, salads and other uncooked vegetables or fruits can be suspect, and if your immune system is particularly fragile, it is perhaps not wise to play that numbers game.

Buffets, including salad bars, are frequently laid out for many hours at a time and are notoriously vulnerable to contamination. This is due not only to their great exposure to air in a place where people are milling about, but also because warm foods are rarely kept hot enough to destroy bacteria but rather at a temperature that encourages their rapid multiplication.

Foods sold from street vendors should be avoided. Though many doubtless are earnestly conscientious in their work, they simply do not have the facilities to assure proper sanitation. The greatest risk (read: not on your life) comes from vendors who cook raw, unprocessed meats (example: for chicken or steak sandwiches), while vendors who handle only fruits are the safest. Again, if your immune system is particularly fragile, none of these should be patronized, including the fruit stands.

When traveling abroad, be mindful that the United States has some of the highest sanitation levels in the world and therefore that you will likely encounter standards that are lower. Especially in Third World countries the difference in standards is apt to be dramatic.

If, while traveling, you are eating out, all of the suggestions above should be followed even more scrupulously. Boil your water before drinking it, or rely on **well-known internationally recognized brands of bottled water.** That water is merely bottled is not a sufficient assurance of safety. The bottled-water industry is barely regulated in this country, some bottled waters coming straight and unfiltered from the municipal water supplies of the bottler. Standards may be much lower as you travel, and it is therefore safest to rely only on international brands of known repute. These well-known brands of bottled waters may be still or sparkling, but if you *must* select a water of local manufacture, choose one that is carbonated. Carbonation makes water sufficiently acidic to kill many microorganisms. In the mid-1970s an outbreak of cholera in Portugal was traced to a bottling plant that bottled both carbonated and noncarbonated waters. The subsequent investigation revealed that only those who had drunk the noncarbonated water were infected.

Less obvious is the ice added to drinks. This is, of course, as potentially harmful as the water from which it is made. Whereas in alcoholic beverages it is possible that the alcohol, when straight and undiluted (for instance, a scotch-on-the-rocks), is sufficient to destroy harmful bacteria, as the ice melts and weakens the alcohol mixture, there comes a time when the alcohol is too dilute and the ice continues to melt, adding more and more pathogens, if present. Better to drink uniced beverages that are cold and avoid those that need icing.

If you are cooking while traveling, fruits and vegetables should be given the extra precaution not only of a thorough washing, but a subsequent brief soak (fifteen to twenty seconds) in mildly chlorinated water (1 tablespoon chlorine bleach to 1 quart water). This is for the dual reasons that the tap water in which you wash the vegetables may not otherwise be sanitary, and also because vegetables grown in other countries are frequently fertilized with raw manure, which can transfer whatever pathogens it may harbor to the fruits and vegetables. Even after taking these precautions it is safest to peel all fruits and thoroughly cook all vegetables.

A handy tip to ward off traveler's diarrhea is to eat a locally produced fermented dairy product, such as yogurt, which is made from pasteurized milk. This will help acclimate your system to strains of local "friendly flora" or "good" bacteria upon which it depends as part of the digestive process. The regional variations of useful bacteria, while not toxic, may be enough to wreak havoc with your gastrointestinal tract until they are assimilated by your body. By introducing them to your system in this manner, much simple traveler's diarrhea may be avoided. More severe and potentially lethal diarrhea (the famous Montezuma's revenge), is due to pathogens which may be avoided following the food-safety guidelines previously outlined.

PART THREE

Dietary
Troubleshooting

Diarrhea

The issues surrounding diarrhea are as sensitive and serious as any might be concerning health and well-being. The loss of bodily control can be demoralizing and contribute to feelings of shame and depression. Diarrhea can potentially lead to rampant weight loss, malabsorption, and a host of other problems such as dehydration, reduced metabolism, chronic dependence on nutritional supplements, and the need for total parenteral nutrition (intravenous feeding). Now is the most important time to work in partnership with your doctor, for diagnosis of the cause or causes of diarrhea can be long and frustrating. Any diarrhea that is severe or prolonged (more than two to three days) should be taken extremely seriously and requires immediate medical attention, for in no other situation is the likelihood of sudden, dramatic weight loss greater. This is also a time when you yourself may have to bring to your treatment regimen certain knowledge and skills that your doctor is simply not equipped to offer.

While not all diarrhea is caused by improper diet, any diarrhea can be greatly worsened or prolonged by eating inappropriately. Diarrhea itself can become something of a self-perpetuating syndrome, where the lining of the bowel becomes so aggravated that its ability to function (that is, to process and absorb food) is compromised. In advanced cases the microvilli (microscopic hairlike extensions of the intestine which give it the vast surface necessary for absorption) can slough off, rendering the gut incapable of performing its function; hence malabsorption.

The dietary management of diarrhea requires a two-pronged approach: you have to avoid the things that will aggravate and prolong the situation and, more proactively, do the things that will actually work toward correcting the problem. However, I must repeat: NOT ALL DIARRHEA IS CAUSED BY OR CAN BE CORRECTED BY DIET ALONE. SEVERE OR PROLONGED DIARRHEA REQUIRES MEDICAL ATTENTION.

The first strategy is, of course, not to expose yourself to any of the many causative agents (toxins, pathogens) that are liable to induce diarrhea in the first place. For this you should carefully review the chapters in Part Two, "Food and Water Safety." To reiterate: much diarrhea, while not caused by diet per se, is the result of food poisoning in varying degrees, or of pathogens introduced into the body via food.

When diarrhea does occur, you must mobilize all of your defense strategies to control it immediately, before it has the opportunity to worsen and self-perpetuate. To attempt to control it by degrees is risky. Making modifications that way may prove too little too late. Significant irritation of the lining of the bowel can occur, which itself may cause the diarrhea to persist. Therefore, **remove the following from your diet immediately:**

FOODS TO AVOID

EXCESSIVE FATS AND OILS

Without question greasy, high-fat, or fried foods should be deleted from the diet. Fats are difficult for your body to digest under the best of circumstances; when you are sick they can cause not only diarrhea, but nausea, gas, and bloating. Fats and oils are a natural laxative, which can speed and facilitate motility (the disgorging of the intestine) and can also interfere with the intestinal tract's ability to absorb food. We all at some time have eaten some greasy food that has left an "oil slick" coating our mouth and tongue. Think of the *Exxon Valdez* oil spill and all of those greasy seagulls that people scrubbed for months. When detergents had done what they could do, the shoreline was peppered with special enzymes to help break down and disperse the oil. Imagine that grease coating your entire intestinal tract and you have an idea of your gut's disadvantage in trying to process the fat and to perform its basic function. The following list provides some examples of foods to avoid most:

Fried foods	Chips	Bacon
Cheesecake	Sausage	Pizza
Tuna in oil	Doughnuts	Mayonnaise

Less obvious, but still quite high in fat content, are:

Gravies	Bologna	Cookies
Peanut butter	Chocolate candies	Hot dogs
Cake	Ice cream	Avocados

WARNING: The "nonfat fat" olestra (brand name Olean) is known to cause severe cramping, diarrhea, and loose stools in many people and to contribute to the malabsorption of many nutrients. It should under no circumstances be eaten.

DAIRY

Most of the world's population never sees milk beyond mother's milk and manages to live quite happily without it. In fact, approximately 70 to 90 percent of the world's population, including infants, are lactose intolerant to some degree. Lactose is a complex sugar occurring only in dairy products (and in all dairy products, including powdered milk), which requires a special enzyme (lactase) in order to be broken down into a form that the body can digest. When this enzyme is not present, lactose sours and ferments in the bowel and can cause not only diarrhea, but also nausea (ranging from slight to extreme malaise), cramping, gas, bloating, and acid stomach.

In infancy our bodies produce lactase as a naturally occurring enzyme. As we grow older and are weaned, our bodies lose the ability to produce this enzyme as we cease to drink milk. This is the standard progression the world over. In America (and some Scandinavian countries), however, the situation is a little different. Americans are among the few people in the world who routinely drink milk into adulthood. This is largely due to the spectacularly successful marketing campaign sponsored by the American Dairy Association in the early part of this century, which established "dairy" as an entire food group. Many Americans, who have regularly downed their daily glass(es) of milk, have artificially prolonged their body's ability to produce lactase and can indeed digest milk and other dairy products with no ill effects. Many more—indeed, the vast majority—have only partly sustained this ability and are therefore lactose intolerant in varying degrees. There are two variables here, and it is important to understand them both:

First, as noted, people are lactose intolerant to varying degrees, some extremely, others only mildly. Most people fit somewhere in the middle and never know they are lactose intolerant at all. Frequently, for example, a person will not recognize that midmorning gas or mild malaise occurs only on days when he has breakfasted on a bowl of cereal with milk or that his indigestion following pizza is not repeated after another meal containing the same amount of fat and spice, but no dairy product. Also, lactose may be tolerated when it is buffered by the concurrent intake of other food. For example, a cup of milk ingested with a bowl of cereal might be tolerated, which, when drunk plain and on an empty stomach, might incur the litany of complaints common to lactose intolerance.

It is remarkable how individual our systems are, and no one but ourselves can judge our degree, if any, of lactose intolerance. Be mindful, however, that even people who are not normally lactose intolerant frequently become so during bouts of diarrhea. It is therefore prudent to discontinue all dairy intake during any episode of gastrointestinal upset, so that lactose intolerance does not exacerbate the problem.

Secondly, lactose is present in inverse proportion to butterfat content. In other words, the degree of intolerance reaction diminishes in dairy products with an increased butterfat content. That is to say; skim milk has more lactose than whole milk, whole milk has more lactose than half-and-half, and so on. Some people find themselves so narrowly defined on the continuum of lactose intolerance that they can eat premium brands of ice cream but not generic or "store" brands, which typically have a lower butterfat content. This second factor of lactose intolerance is less relevant to the problem of diarrhea, than is the problem of fat intake discussed before. It is included here to promote a more thorough understanding of dairy/lactose issues, and for its application to other problems in which diarrhea is not present (nausea, for example). Further, fermented dairy products (including aged cheeses, yogurt, buttermilk, and kefir) have all had their lactose greatly reduced by bacterial action. Fermentation functions in much the same way as lactase to break down the lactose into forms that the body can digest. In parts of the world where dairy consumption continues into adulthood, it is almost entirely in this form.

There are several options for people who are lactose intolerant, in addition to the above-mentioned fermented dairy products. "Sweet acidophilus" or "lactose-reduced" milks (so marked on the label) are both possibilities. Sweet acidophilus is a nonsour-tasting strain of the bacteria used to ferment yogurt, so that in fact this milk is actually fermented, although its taste is the same as that of standard milk. Lactose-reduced milk is milk dosed with the same enzyme your body has lost its ability to produce (lactase), which has proceeded to break down the lactose into the simple sugar that your body can absorb. Your palate is also able to perceive the sugar in its simpler form though the milk actually has no increased sugar content.

The enzyme lactase is further available to you in pill and liquid form under the brand names Lactaid and Dairy Ease (however, it should be noted that Dairy Ease contains mannitol, which can produce diarrheal problems of its own—see the paragraph on sugar substitutes on page 81). To use this product, add some drops to any liquid dairy product and allow it to stand a prescribed length of time, usually overnight, while the enzyme action breaks down the lactose. Alternatively, the pill form can be taken shortly before eating any sort of dairy product and the enzyme action takes place in the digestive tract as it normally would. These excellent products are completely natural, widely available (in most drugstores and many grocery stores), and work well for many, but not all, people. Only by trying them yourself to determine your individual response can you know their efficacy in relation to your own degree of lactose intolerance and personal constitution.

Another option is the soy- or rice-based milk substitutes, such as EdenSoy, which are becoming increasingly available in grocery stores. Some of these beverages combine soy and rice to provide a complementary (complete) protein. While not a complete nutritional substitute for actual milk, they are acceptable substitutes for people who are lactose intolerant. Even if you should find that you do not care for their taste as a beverage, do not overlook their uses as an accompaniment to breakfast cereal or as the base for a lactose-free blender drink. For many cooking purposes the substitution will go virtually unnoticed.

Lest you be led astray by the above-mentioned considerations, let me reiterate here: During any bout of diarrhea it is much safer to remove dairy products from your diet completely for the duration of the episode. THIS INCLUDES FOODS MADE WITH SUBSTANTIAL

PROPORTIONS OF MILK PRODUCTS, such as puddings or milk gravies. Products marked "Parve" contain no dairy products.

Note: "Dairy" is strictly the "fruit of the breast." It does not include eggs, coconut "milk," nondairy creamers, or any of the other things that are either lumped into the "fourth food group" or are given names based on their similarities to true dairy products. Only actual milk and milk by-products and derivatives contain lactose.

HIGH-CONCENTRATION SUGAR
(ALSO, ALCOHOL, PROTEIN POWDERS, AND SUGAR SUBSTITUTES)

Sugar is a substance, like alcohol, that is hydroscopic or "water seeking." They both have the power to literally pull from your system sufficient water to cause dehydration (discussed more fully under "Fluids," on page 87). This is the famous "dry-mouth" associated with hangovers. It is also why a bowl of ice cream or a chocolate bar will leave you thirsty. In normal circumstances the digestive tract can absorb the sugar quickly enough so that nothing more than a glass or two of water is necessary to correct the temporary dehydration. During an episode of diarrhea, however, the gut, with its diminished ability to function, can neither absorb nor disgorge the sugar quickly enough to prevent dehydration. This can also possibly initiate watery bowel syndrome, a situation in which large enough quantities of water swiftly reach the gut to trigger the loose stools associated with diarrhea. This is another instance of how diarrhea can begin to self-perpetuate even when the original causative agent may no longer be a factor. Too often, people rely on sugary soft drinks, drink mixes, and the like for their fluid intake, or will eat bowl after bowl of ice cream, thinking that the blandness will suit them, when actually they are actively contributing to the persistence of the problem.

Slightly different in their action, but producing similar results, high-protein powders—sold generally as weight-gain products for weight-lifters—can also be guilty of fostering watery bowel syndrome, for in their intense concentration they, too, are hydroscopic. Even under normal circumstances their value is questionable (see "Protein," under Chapter 2), but in episodes of diarrhea they should be avoided entirely.

Last, beware of dietetic versions of foods. Many sugar substitutes, most notably sorbitol or mannitol (both natural sweeteners), can cause intolerance reactions of their own, prominent among them diarrhea. These substitutes are found not only in many diet drinks, sugar-free chewing gums, and dietetic candies, but also in virtually every major brand of toothpaste, where they contribute to flavor and also, by their hydroscopic nature, keep the paste moist. Tartar Control Dental Care, by the Arm & Hammer company, is a brand that does not contain sorbitol. Alternatively, baking soda may be used harmlessly and effectively throughout an episode of diarrheal illness.

CAFFEINE

All of us know and most of us love caffeine. It is present as an additive in many foods besides coffee and tea, its most familiar forms. Chocolate contains significant amounts of caffeine, which, even when not in a high-fat, high-sugar form, would make it suspect during a spell of diarrhea. So do many soft drinks, notably colas.

Caffeine's detrimental actions during episodes of diarrhea are twofold and as follows:

First, caffeine functions as a diuretic, which, in a high-caffeine beverage like coffee, causes more fluid loss than intake. Though the diuretic effect is, of course, diminished as the concentration of caffeine is reduced, the effect is still present and should be guarded against, as dehydration is a potentially lethal consequence of diarrhea (see "Fluids," on page 87).

Secondly, caffeine can stimulate contractions of the bowel, which in turn can worsen diarrhea. This is true with caffeine in any form, but is particularly noticeable with coffee, famous for its laxative effect. With coffee there is an additional phenomenon: it stimulates the secretion of gastric acids, which can in turn exacerbate diarrhea and acid stomach. This is true not only of regular coffee, but also of decaffeinated and acid-neutralized coffees.

If you are a person who cannot bear the thought of morning without a hot caffeine beverage, the suggestion here is to switch your allegiance to tea, preferably weak. While this is primarily because weak tea has, of course, less caffeine, the tannins in tea have a mild constipating effect that tends to counterbalance the effect of the caffeine. (*Note:* teas drunk with milk will not have the same effect, as the milk will bind with the tannins and circumvent this action.) Beware, however, of noncaffeine grain beverages (such as Postum), which are frequently recommended as substitutes for coffee. They can have strong laxative effects of their own, as can many herbal tisanes (teas), and are best avoided. Of the latter, tisanes made with aloe leaves or senna are among the worst offenders commonly available.

INDIGESTIBLES
(INCLUDING SPICES, CRUCIFEROUS VEGETABLES, AND LEGUMES)

Some varieties of foods are more difficult to digest than others and therefore present an even greater challenge to the digestive tract under stress.

Spices, with their heavy aromatic oils, include not only the fiery hot peppers and chilis that we associate with "spicy" foods, but also commonplace spices like allspice, cinnamon, clove, pepper, and nutmeg. This last group, in mild concentration, usually presents no problem, but when used heavily or frequently can overtax the intestinal tract.

Cruciferous vegetables are those in the large cabbage family, well known for their ability to cause gas in many people. Broccoli, Brussels sprouts, cabbage, cauliflower, and onions are all members of this family. Because of their high sulfur-compound content and high insoluble-fiber content, they are among the most difficult items in a standard diet to digest.

Legumes (peas and beans) are difficult for the average digestion under normal circumstances. Even more famous than cabbage for their gas-causing qualities, they are also extremely high in insoluble fiber content (discussed at greater length on page 84). Their most concentrated form is in dried and reconstituted foods such as bean soups and baked or refried beans, all of which should be avoided during episodes of diarrhea.

CARBONATION

Carbonated beverages, including seltzer and sparkling mineral waters, do not aggravate diarrhea but in certain people can increase the stomach cramping that sometimes goes along with it. If you should find this to be the case, it would be wise to discontinue carbonated beverages until cramping stops. See notes on carbonation under "Nausea" (Chapter 11) and "Eating Defensively Away from Home" (Chapter 9).

INSOLUBLE FIBER

Insoluble dietary fiber is that part of plants which we cannot digest and which passes through our bowels relatively intact. Though it contains no nutrients per se, it is a very necessary part of our digestive process. Among other things, fiber largely makes up the vehicle that moves nutrient-bearing food through our digestive tract, and it speeds motility. In this form—as insoluble fiber—it was formerly referred to as "roughage" or even "nature's broom." As the typical American diet is unduly heavy in fats and meats (which contain no fiber), this action of fiber is what has most frequently been cultivated as an antidote for constipation. Such is the action of insoluble fiber. But there is another type of fiber as different from it as night to day, and it is soluble fiber, explained on page 85.

FOODS AND PRACTICES THAT PROMOTE RECOVERY AND HEALING

> It must be stressed that medical intervention is necessary to determine and manage many of the causes of diarrhea, and until these causative factors are corrected, the episode may continue and worsen. With any diarrhea that is severe or lasts more than three days, consult your health-care provider immediately.

SOLUBLE FIBER

One hears a great deal about fiber as an American dietary concern, that we don't get enough and that we all need more. True as this may be for the general population, it is a vast oversimplification of the issue. Lack of understanding about fiber can rob you of your greatest potential dietary ally in combating and reversing diarrhea.

Soluble fiber is the gum, pectin, and mucilage of plant material, and its action in our digestive tract is quite different from that of insoluble fiber. With its ability to absorb water and expand, it functions to bind together the contents of the intestine, providing a very valuable assist toward controlling the loose stools typical of diarrhea. Observe how a bowl of oatmeal, grits, or cream of wheat congeals as it cools, an action that is not dissimilar to what happens in the gut. This binding process has the potential to provide the greatest relief from diarrhea short of drug intervention, and sometimes it provides relief where drug intervention fails.

Dietary modifications are meant not to replace drug therapies but to enhance their success. At the least, to undergo drug therapy for diarrhea but to continue to eat quantities of insoluble fiber is to undermine your treatment. To focus on soluble and delete insoluble fiber will greatly enhance the efficacy of any drug therapy prescribed.

Most fruits and vegetables contain both forms of fiber. Your goal is to eat only the soluble and avoid the insoluble. Generally and simply stated, insoluble fiber is the outer covering of things and soluble fiber is the inside "flesh" or pulp of things. For example: the inside or "flesh" of a baked potato is soluble fiber. The potato skin is insoluble fiber. During a bout of diarrhea you would want to eat only the inside of the potato (mashed potatoes are excellent) and discard the skins. The same is true with apples: the flesh of an apple, raw or cooked (applesauce) is an excellent source of soluble fiber. The peel, which is high in insoluble fiber, should not be eaten. Perhaps an easy way to remember this is to think of the banana: the inside of a banana is another excellent source of soluble fiber, while the peel is so insolubly fibrous that even the average garbage disposal cannot handle it.

Let's look at some more examples: White rice and brown rice are actually the same rice. Brown rice has had only some of its outer covering (the bran) removed, while white rice has had it all removed. Therefore, white rice is the soluble-fiber part of the grain with the insoluble part—the bran—removed. The same with wheat: whole wheat is that in which the bran has been milled with the rest of the grain and hence contains the insoluble fiber. White bread is made with just that part of the grain which is soluble fiber.

If you use this consideration of inside versus outside, you can determine for yourself in most cases whether a particular food consists of soluble or insoluble fiber. For instance: Are leafy green vegetables, like lettuce, high in soluble or insoluble fiber? Ever try to peel a lettuce leaf? It's almost all "outside," therefore, it's almost all insoluble. It should be noted, however, that most seeds (including nuts and corn products), though contained in shells or husks, are high in insoluble fiber.

Please do not assume from the discussion above that the outer coverings of things are not generally good nutritionally. Indeed, many vitamins and minerals are also contained in these superficial coverings. However, the urgency and seriousness of diarrhea makes it well worthwhile to delete them from the diet for the duration of the episode. After the problem of diarrhea is corrected, they form an important component of a well-rounded diet.

FLUIDS

Dehydration is a potentially lethal consequence of diarrhea. Sixty percent of the AIDS-related admissions to San Francisco General Hospital result from such dehydration. No other single fact of diet is more important at this time than maintaining your fluid intake. It is impossible to overemphasize the importance of this. Water is by far your body's most essential component and its loss affects its very ability to function. However, when fluids are flushed from our bodies, more·than just water is expelled. Water-soluble vitamins and electrolytes are also lost at an alarming rate. This is in part why a bout of diarrhea is so exhausting: Our body's ability to absorb any nutrients from food on its swift passage through our digestive tract is greatly reduced even when the actual problem of malabsorption does not exist. Therefore it is greatly desired that the fluids we drink be not merely nutrient bearing, but also rich in those substances which are so rapidly being stripped from our bodies.

Optimal Replacement Fluids

Electrolytes (chloride, potassium, and sodium) are chemicals necessary for the delicate chemical/electrical functioning of our bodies. Without these water-soluble substances we feel listless and tired. Diuretics, excessive perspiration, vomiting, and diarrhea can all flush them from our systems. Their replacement is essential not only to health but also to feelings of well-being and vitality. "Sports beverages" are the most efficient mechanism generally available for the rapid replacement of electrolytes. These have been designed expressly for the purpose. With their carefully balanced osmalality (the optimal viscosity of fluids necessary to enhance absorption) they are literally absorbed even more quickly than water. Gatorade, the first and still most widely

NECTAR "SPORTS DRINK"
2 cups water (or rice water, see below)
2 cups apricot, peach, or pear nectar
1 tsp. salt
1 tsp. baking soda
2 Tbs. sugar

(or 2 Tbs. corn syrup)

HOMEMADE "SPORTS DRINK"
1 quart water (or rice water, see below)
1 tsp. salt
1 tsp. baking soda
¼ cup sugar

(or ¼ cup corn syrup)
1 Tbs. Kool-Aid-type drink mix

This recipe will provide chloride, sodium, and carbohydrates, but not potassium, unless it is blended with a banana (an excellent source not only of potassium but also of soluble fiber). Of course, a banana could also be eaten along with this beverage.

CAUTION: The use of over-the-counter potassium-tablet supplements to make up the balance is not advised unless prescribed by a physician, for not only is their absorption in this form unsure during episodes of diarrhea, but their concentrated form can be extremely harsh on the stomach. Soluble potassium supplements are available only by prescription.

available of these, was designed to meet the needs of athletes who, in Florida summer training, would flush away vast quantities of sodium and potassium, in addition to water, through perspiration. The beverage also contains calorie-bearing carbohydrates in the form of a low concentration of sugar, as a ready source of energy. Gatorade is available in both a bottled form and a powdered drink-mix form, which is valuable to keep on hand and less expensive than the bottled version.

Though formulas for dehydration in infants (Infalyte and Pedialyte) have long been marketed, only recently has there been one specifically designed for adults. BestLyte, made by the Choose Health company ([800] 757-6339), is designed specifically for people living with AIDS who are experiencing dehydration due to diarrhea or vomiting. In addition to being an electrolyte-repletion formula, it is made with a high percentage of rice syrup solids, which have been shown to slow motility.

It is possible to make homemade versions of a "sports drink," though including the important potassium component is not especially easy. Apricot, peach, and pear nectars (in that rapidly descending order) are rich in potassium and are therefore ideal choices to use. In an occasional individual these fruit nectars will actually increase diarrhea (you will note the conspicuous absence of prune juice from the list), in which instance it should certainly be discontinued. Some fine day, when the sun is shining and all is right with the world, you might try one of these nectars to determine in advance whether or not it affects you this way. If it does, better to opt for one of the other electrolyte-repletion beverages described in this chapter.

If there is a single, handy piece of advice in this book, it is that you should use these "sports drinks" for fluid replacement during episodes of diarrhea. Time and again, after I have recommended their use to people in the throes of debilitating diarrhea, the recovered feeling of well-being has been astonishing. It goes far toward restoring vitality, the loss of which is one of the most devastating consequences of diarrhea.

> ## HORCHATA
> 1 part white rice, preferably short grain
>   rice such as River Rice
> 4 parts water
>
> Boil rice in water until tender. Strain off water and allow
> to cool. Rice water may be sweetened slightly if desired.
> Have the rice with dinner.

The rice-syrup solids mentioned above are the soluble-fiber component of rice and have a basis in Hispanic folk medicine which you may put to good use. *Horchata* is a rice-water beverage that may be drunk by itself or used in any of the "sports beverage" recipes and will simultaneously offer hydration and soluble fiber to assist in binding the stool.

Other fluids, too, are valuable for supplying nutrients which water cannot provide. Fruit juices are ideally suited for this, as they are lactose free, nutrient bearing, and easy to digest. To aid in digestion many of the thicker juices, such as apricot nectar, are best diluted with water up to 50 percent. This not only makes them more palatable for many people, but also decreases their osmalality. Citrus or tomato juices, while excellent sources of potassium, have a great enough acid content to cause stomach distress for many people. Should this be the case for you, try very dilute solutions or simply avoid them.

Finally, thirst is not a completely accurate guide to the need for fluid intake, as thirst is frequently slaked before all depleted fluids have been restored. With any bout of diarrhea, fluid loss may be assumed. Aim for drinking about a cup of repletion formula or other liquid per bowel movement. Constant steady sipping is preferable to overwhelming the digestive tract with sudden great quantities of fluid, for the overload itself can serve to stress the system and exacerbate the diarrhea.

ANTIBIOTICS AND DIARRHEA

One of the principal mechanisms in the digestion of food is the bacterial action by which foodstuffs are broken down into simpler components. Without the action of this "friendly flora" of the gut, our bodies cannot digest and absorb the foods we eat. The action of an antibiotic is to clean the system of all foreign bacteria—both infectious and friendly. When this happens, the digestive tract is left with food in an unprocessed state it cannot absorb and diarrhea is frequently the result. To avoid this it is necessary to replace the "good" bacteria on a regular basis while taking any course of antibiotics. Fortunately, this is a simple matter of eating or drinking any fermented dairy product that has a live culture, such as yogurt, buttermilk, kefir (a fermented milk a little like yogurt), or sweet acidophilus milk. This will quickly reestablish the desired colony of bacteria and diminish antibiotic-induced diarrhea, usually quite dramatically. Be advised, however, that the antibiotic will continue to eradicate this newly reestablished colony. It is necessary to continue eating the yogurt or buttermilk on a daily basis until several days after the medication is finished, due to the residual effects of the medicine remaining in your system. Yogurt, buttermilk, kefir, and sweet acidophilus milk are the most reliable sources of the needed live culture, and need not be consumed in any great quantities: several tablespoons or ounces twice a day should be sufficient. Processed cheeses contain no active cultures and aged cheeses contain them in widely varying degrees, depending not only on type of cheese but also on age and condition. For those who are lactose intolerant or who wish, for other reasons, to avoid dairy, acidophilus supplements are available in most health-food- and many drugstores and will answer the purpose admirably. Some are even compounded with citrus pectin (a soluable fiber) to aid in binding the stool. Ask your pharmacist.

BRATT DIET

BRATT is the acronym for the diet routinely recommended for people with diarrhea, and stands for Bananas, Rice, Applesauce, and Tea and Toast. You can deduce from our discussions so far the nutritive contribution of each component: bananas, (white) rice, applesauce, and (white bread) toast are all sources of soluble fiber. Bananas replace lost potassium, and tea, with its mild constipating effect, replaces lost fluid. All these components are lactose free and virtually fat free, assuming you eat your toast dry and drink your tea without milk. Skip putting jam or jelly on the toast, as these are too high in sugar. There is no special magic to the BRATT elements, and you may freely substitute other foods that fall within these same guidelines.

CHEWING THOROUGHLY

This advice is just as simple as it sounds, yet frequently it is either taken for granted or ignored, so that the admonition is rarely made to adults. Chewing is the first mechanism of our digestion and one of the most important. Unlike some other animals, we have no elaborate grinding mechanism (such as a gizzard) farther down, and therefore the entire remainder of our digestive tract is at a disadvantage if we overlook this preliminary. Digestion itself even begins with the enzymes in the mouth. One of the kindest, and certainly the simplest, things you can do for your digestive tract in all circumstances, but certainly during episodes of diarrhea, is to chew your food thoroughly.

CONTINUE EATING

Many people believe that a time of fasting is an appropriate response to diarrhea, in order to "rest the bowel." Though this can seemingly address symptoms, fasting not only deprives the body of nutrition, but does nothing corrective to address the problem. Eating appropriate foods, such as low-fat, soluble-fiber, dairy-free foods in small, frequent meals with an adequate intake of fluids will go much farther toward maintaining adequate nutrition and will offer the greatest dietary assist possible to restoring the bowel to normalcy.

NUTRITIONAL SUPPLEMENTS

Liquid nutritional supplements can be extremely valuable during episodes of diarrhea. They are basically predigested food, ready for your gut to absorb, and are available in any drug and many grocery stores. With their scientifically designed formulas of modified fatty acid chains, they will be absorbed if any nutrient can be. A variety are commercially available, including Advera, which is specifically designed to accommodate the needs of people with AIDS. Their greatest drawbacks are their cost and their taste. (For recipes to "jazz up" nutritional supplements, see Part Four).

THOROUGH RINSING

Soap and detergents can both be powerful laxatives and many people fail to rinse their dishes properly. (Many times while running a kitchen staffed with volunteers I would see dishes set in a drainboard to dry still cascading soap bubbles.) Ingested on a regular basis, the residue can contribute needlessly to diarrhea. This contributing factor can easily be avoided simply by rinsing all dishes, pots, and pans until no soap remains.

BUTT KINDNESS

Rectal irritation is, of course, quite common in times of sustained diarrhea, but there are ways in which it can be minimized.

You may find that moistening your toilet paper will significantly reduce the irritation of frequent wiping. Any mild, unscented hand lotion, such as Lubriderm, will help. Moistening tissue with witch hazel, which is a mild astringent, will soothe irritation that already exists and may be used in alternation. Finally, soaking in a warm, not hot, tub or sitz bath with baking soda or Epsom salts can further soothe the outraged bottom.

Diarrhea can be one of the most demoralizing aspects of AIDS or any other illness. The loss of bodily control, the invasion of private space if we need assistance, the sheer exhaustion, the mess, all these factors can contribute to feelings of shame and a weakening of our resolve to go on living. Yet human dignity resides in more than bodily function and absence of social awkwardnesses. Services that we would gladly perform for a loved one may seem too much to ask for ourselves as we perhaps question our own worth. I encourage the reader to carefully think through these issues and to be kind to yourself in these matters. As commitment to living is an identifying characteristic of long-term survivors of AIDS, it is best to have grounded your feelings and commitment, so that unexpected emotions do not take you unaware.

RECIPE SUGGESTIONS
- Egg drop soup
- Avgolemono
- Chicken and dumplings
- Shrimp pie
- Orange glazed chicken
- Ginger sherry pork chops

ᕮᨆᕭ **11**

Nausea

Nausea affects many people while they are sick. Rather than simply being a problem of discomfort (a reasonable quality-of-life issue in its own right), nausea can so interfere with the desire and ability to eat that it becomes a cause of malnourishment itself. While nausea can be the result of sickness or of various drug therapies, it is triggered most frequently through our senses of smell and taste. Learning to manage trigger situations and our responses to them can frequently circumvent a pattern of ever-worsening reactions. These reactions, if not checked, can lead from decreased appetite at its mildest to revulsion against all food at its worst.

Severe, chronic nausea should not be taken lightly, and your physician may be able to assist you with medications to relieve it. There are, however, many ways in which you can minimize the possibility of its onset by changes in routine and diet.

THE SUBJECTIVE RESPONSE

Different stimuli make different people nauseous, and it is important to listen carefully to our own promptings as to what may suit us, as taste is an extremely subjective response. This does not, however, mean that it is wise to rely on our favorite foods to still "taste good" to us. In fact, the reverse can be true. It is possible to set up an association between times of nausea and certain foods. When associations are created, those foods can later trigger a nausea response, possibly spoiling our love for foods we have always enjoyed.

It is important to consider carefully what foods might best suit us when we are nauseous. Most often for most people, that means soft, mild foods. But again, this is a subjective consideration and frequently conventional thinking such as "Bland foods are best" can simply break down. To illustrate: For most people, fiery, hot, spicy food sounds like the worst possible choice during a bout of nausea, but for a small group of people (the author among them), it is what is most apt to quell episodes of nausea. (This is because the capsicum in chilies can stimulate the flow of gastric juices and awaken the appetite enough to overcome nausea.) This example about spicy/hot foods is not made as a suggestion (unless it should sound good to you and you have avoided them in deference to "conventional wisdom"), but to illustrate that you should eat what foods best suit you, even if that means a diet of candy bars and anchovies. THE IMPORTANT THING IS TO CONTINUE EATING BY EATING WHATEVER YOU *CAN* EAT.

THE SMELL RESPONSE

Our sense of taste is intimately bound up in our ability to smell. The old saying that if you can't smell something you can't taste it is very nearly true. The standard experiment to prove this is to chop some apple and some onion to a similarly fine dice and to have someone who is holding her nose taste one of them "blindfolded." In most cases the person will not know for a while which she is tasting. The breakdown in this example comes when the volatile fragrance oils reach our noses through the "back door" where our sinuses open to our palates.

In times of nausea, if we reduce the odor of food (or our exposure to it), we will frequently reduce our visceral and negative response to food. There are a number of simple ways in which this may be accomplished.

The first method is to absent yourself from food odors as much as possible, which in many cases means that you should avoid cooking aromas. Make a strategy. Try to cook in advance for a meal later, possibly taking a walk in the fresh air after cooking, to clear your head. A slow cooker, such as a Crock-Pot, if isolated in such a way that the cooking odors do not permeate your living area, can be very helpful. As you cook, keep as much fresh air circulating as is reasonably possible. In the winter, when indoor air can become choked with stale cooking odors, open a window and put on a sweater. During a time of nausea "convenience foods" that are simply heated and eaten can be of their greatest value, not so much for their ease in preparation as for the fact that they largely absent you from the cooking process and attendant odors. If you have a friend or family member who can cook for you, so much the better. This may be the time to take advantage of a friendly neighbor or co-worker's offer to "do something." In an ideal situation the cooking would be done out of your presence so that the cooking odors don't trigger nausea responses even before the food arrives.

Another method is to eat cold food. The fragrance oils that give food its odor are not so volatile when cold; hence the same food has dramatically less scent. Think of cold roast chicken versus hot roast chicken. Chicken salad, pasta salad, cheese, peanut butter— the list of cold or room-temperature foods goes on and on (for particular recipes, see Part Four). As most cold foods are hot foods first, again, try to cook in advance for a meal later. Consider picking up that chicken already roasted, putting it in the refrigerator as soon as you get home and making chicken salad when it is cold.

Though there are many delicious cold foods, chances are that if nausea is an ongoing problem, you will tire of them. In eating hot meals, fresh air can again come to your rescue. We have all heard of various ways to peel or chop onions without tears (holding a match in our front teeth, cutting the onion under running water, et cetera). The only method I know that really, *really* works is to have a fan to the left or right blowing the fumes away before they have a chance to reach your face. This method also can be used when eating a hot meal. Preventing the fragrance of warm food from wafting up into your face can make an enormous difference. Sitting beside an open window while eating can also serve this purpose, as can taking your meals outdoors.

HELPFUL GRAVITY

Gravity can work for or against you in assuring that which goes down does not come back up. In times of sickness, eating in bed is common. Sitting up, even if in bed, for an hour after eating will greatly reduce the chances of food backing up into your esophagus and stimulating a taste/response that can lead to nausea and gagging.

LIQUIDS

Drinking just before or while you eat can, not surprisingly, make what is in your stomach more fluid, increasing the chances of the same reflux action described above. Avoid drinking for about an hour before, during, and at least twenty minutes after eating. This will greatly reduce the danger of setting up a taste/gag response. The less fluid are the contents of the stomach, the less likely they are to "slosh" back up. Eating dry foods, such as crackers, toast, or cereal can also help achieve this same goal. When drinking, sip slowly. Using a straw may help.

For some people the clean, clear tastelessness of club soda, seltzer, or mineral water is very soothing; others are bothered by the carbonation and find that "flat" soft drinks suit them better, as belching or a bloated feeling may result from the gas. This is a matter of personal choice. (See note under "Ginger" on page 99). At any rate, clear liquids are frequently better tolerated. Acidic fruit juices, particularly citrus or tomato, can be especially irritating unless very dilute. Coffee, including decaffeinated and acid-neutralized coffees, can cause a drop in the pressure in the esophagus. This, in turn, allows the contents of the stomach to come back up into the throat, offering again the reflux action that sets in motion the taste/gag response.

If nausea is extreme, dehydration can result from continued vomiting. Should this occur, the danger of electrolyte depletion exists. For appropriate electrolyte repletion beverages, see page 87.

GINGER

The long folk tradition of eating ginger to quell nausea is borne out by research, and unlike many medicines, it has no side effects. In fact, taken in dosages of one half gram, it has frequently shown greater efficacy than standard antiemetic (antinausea) drugs such as Dramamine. While ginger capsules may be found in health-food and some drugstores, there is sufficient ginger in ginger ale or gingersnap cookies to quell mild nausea. Stronger doses may be found in ginger beer (which is nonalcoholic) and crystallized ginger candy.

SALT

Salting your food more than you usually do should help quell nausea. Salted crackers, canned soups or broths (usually high in salt), and any foods to which you can pleasantly add a perceptible taste of salt may help reduce feelings of malaise.

INDIGESTIBLES

Fried, greasy, or very fatty foods are difficult to digest and can contribute to feelings of malaise and nausea, and should therefore be avoided. Many common spices such as pepper or nutmeg are also difficult to digest. Flavor interest in food can frequently be achieved by substituting herbs such as basil or parsley, which, with fewer heavy aromatic oils, are easier to digest. Dairy products, for the vast majority of people who are (unknowingly) lactose intolerant, are a common source of nausea, and their deletion from the diet can frequently correct ongoing intermittent nausea. (For a more complete discussion of lactose intolerance, see "Dairy," page 77.) Finally, intensely sweet foods or beverages can precipitate nausea in many people and should be avoided if you find this to be your response.

Severe or chronic nausea, which can be the result of illness, anxiety, chemotherapy, or medication, should be regarded as a serious health problem and discussed with your doctor as such. Antiemetic drugs can be of great help and should be taken at the onset of nausea, before the problem becomes severe. If your standard medications should cause nausea as a side effect, discuss with your doctor changing their schedule (e.g., taking them after meals rather than before, et cetera).

In any case of illness it is of great importance to continue eating. Here is a schedule in sequence of tactics you may try in times of severest nausea:

1. Keep the room cool rather than warm and the air as fresh as possible.

2. When even sipping cool water is not tolerated, try holding a small amount of crushed ice in your mouth and "sipping" at this as it melts. Sitting up will help not only to reduce the chance of choking, but may also reduce the "floating" feeling that can sometimes accompany nausea.

3. When crushed ice is tolerated, try a Popsicle. You may make these yourself using flat ginger ale or diluted fruit juices. These natural flavors are frequently tolerated better than the synthetic flavors of most commercially made Popsicles. If nausea and vomiting have been sufficient to cause dehydration, a "sports drink" such as Gatorade or BestLyte can be frozen into Popsicles and

will help restore lost electrolytes and carbohydrates. (For a more complete discussion of this issue, see "Fluids" on page 86.)

4. When flavored frozen fluids and liquids are tolerated, try gelatins. Again, when homemade with fruit juices, their fresher flavor is more apt to be accepted. "Sports drinks" may also be used as a base for gelatins, as can broths, both of which can supply a certain amount of helpful, nausea-quelling salt. (For gelatin recipes, see Part Four.)

5. As you begin to bridge into semisolid foods, try saltine crackers with sips of whatever soups may appeal to you. The saltiness of canned broths is to your advantage here, as is the fact that their brief heating produces only a slight cooking odor. Consider cold soup if it appeals to you and is available.

6. Fresh fruit, with its "clear" flavors and slight fragrance, is frequently tolerated when savory or sweet flavors are not. It may be eaten chilled and lightly salted. This step may be substituted for number 5, above, depending on your preference.

7. As your appetite returns, you may find that you are very hungry indeed. Try not to overwhelm yourself with eating, which could reprecipitate nausea. Instead, eat small meals with rests in between. Be guided by your own tastes now.

RECIPE SUGGESTIONS
- Avgolemono
- Egg drop soup
- Ginger sherry pork chops
- Baked custard
- Cheesecake
- Chicken and dumplings
- Gingersnaps
- Fruit gelatin

 oran 12

Oral Problems
Including Mouth Soreness, Dry Mouth, and Thrush

Oral problems may result from a host of causes, including thrush, Kaposi's sarcoma lesions, herpes zoster ulcers, and dental problems. Far from being a matter of simple discomfort, any of these conditions can foster an avoidance of eating, which can contribute to serious malnutrition. Again, as in other areas of health concern relating to diet or food intake, consultation with your doctor (and dentist) may provide relieving medical therapy. When oral pain inhibits eating, a localized numbing medication can sometimes provide relief for a length of time sufficient for a meal to be eaten. Concurrently, modifications in diet to accommodate pain and discomfort will allow you the greatest relief. Other suggestions for mouth soreness follow:

THRUSH

Thrush is runaway candida-yeast activity in the mouth, which can alter the mouth's environment sufficiently to cause changes ranging from altered taste perception to severe discomfort, thereby reducing pleasure in food and thus contributing to diminished appetite. Fortunately, thrush is very effectively controlled in most cases by standard prescribed medications. If for some reason they should not be effective in your case (or if you elect to forgo the medication), thrush may be kept to a minimum by reducing the presence in the mouth of the sugars upon which the yeast feeds. If you do have thrush, in addition to scrupulously following the oral hygiene regimen described below, it is important to avoid sugary foods, including candies, desserts, and pastries, sugared breakfast cereals, and soft drinks, all of which can leave a sugar residue in the mouth. As carbohydrates (starches) are rapidly converted to sugars by the enzymes in the mouth, brushing (or at least thorough rinsing) after every meal and snack is important. Dairy products, too, contain lactose, a natural sugar. Frequent rinsing even in the intervals between eating is helpful to maintain the freshness of the mouth.

> **Simple rinsing with a saline solution will help maintain mouth freshness. One teaspoon salt to a quart of water will provide adequate salinity, though you may find that up to a teaspoon of salt to a glass of water provides greater soothing. In this greater concentration a subsequent rinse with fresh plain water will help assure that the salt does not contribute to mouth dryness.**

ORAL HYGIENE

This, of course, begins by working with your dentist to ensure optimal dental health. Assuming that, here are some suggestions for oral health:

Even when your gums are sore, their maintenance is important. Brushing should be done with the softest brush available, which may be made softer still by being rinsed thoroughly in very hot water immediately before use. Keep your toothbrush sanitary by storing it with the head submerged in rubbing alcohol (rinse before using) and replacing it monthly. If it is still too abrasive, try using a cotton swab or a disposable foam stick (a product designed for this purpose and available in many drugstores or hospital-supply stores). If your tongue is not too sore, brush it also. Avoid commercial mouthwashes if they cause discomfort, using instead a mild solution of hydrogen peroxide (mixed 1 part peroxide to 1 part water). Be certain to swish it thoroughly throughout the mouth, including the back molar area, hold it long enough that the foaming action has a chance to work (do not swallow the solution), and follow with a thorough rinse of plain water. Avoid the use of water-shooting "toothbrushes." Be certain that your vitamin C intake is adequate (at least 500 mg per day), as lack of vitamin C is frequently the cause of bleeding gums.

SOFT FOODS

When your mouth is sore, it hurts to chew. A diet of soft foods can probably help. This is referred to as a "soft mechanical diet" for the simple reason that the softness of the food reduces the "mechanics" of chewing, thereby reducing painful friction. Many foods, such as mashed potatoes, cream or egg-drop soups, yogurt, gelatin, and ice cream, are all, by their nature, soft. Meal-like blender drinks can offer great nutritional intake (see Part Four for recipe suggestions). Commercial baby foods, with their wide menu range, may also be useful. Many more foods, indeed virtually all, can be made soft with the aid of a food processor, blender, hand blender, meat grinder, or heavy-duty juicer. (For this latter only certain models, such as the Champion juicer, are appropriate, as the action required is one of grinding and extruding.) Pureeing your own foods has the additional advantage of allowing you to eat those foods that you normally prefer, albeit in a different form. You may add liquid while pureeing your foods so that they may be drunk from a cup or even sipped through a large straw. If you desire additional flavoring, try adding broth or other flavored liquids to dilute the purees. (For a discussion of canned liquid nutritional supplements, see page 93.)

When you become able to eat food with some lumps, try macaroni and cheese, scrambled eggs, oatmeal, cottage cheese, and the softer, spreadable tuna or chicken salads. Stews and heartier soups are also appropriate here, as are softer casseroles. Choose foods in gravies or cream sauces. Moisten drier foods by soaking or dunking them in liquids and sip at an accompanying beverage frequently. Cut meats and other foods into small pieces. While many fruits, such as bananas and avocados, are soft and therefore appropriate, avoid those with a high acid content, such as citrus or tomato, whose acidity is apt to irritate. Vegetables should be cooked until soft. Avoid crunchy foods, such as raw apples or celery.

For some people, certain smooth, soft foods are deceptively difficult to eat and swallow. Peanut butter leaps to mind. Less obvious are very slippery foods such as noodles in a very liquid sauce. Only you can gauge whether these foods are difficult for you. In all of these instances very spicy or acid foods (such as those containing tomatoes) can unduly irritate your mouth and should therefore be avoided. Many times herbal flavorings, such as basil or thyme, are better tolerated and can add interest to foods in lieu of spices such as pepper, curry, or chili powder.

HOT VERSUS COLD FOODS

Physical heat as well as chemical heat (spice) can cause irritation, and therefore room-temperature and chilled foods will be found the most comfortable. For room-temperature foods considerations of food safety come into play (see Part Two on safe food-handling practices). It is important that foods not merely be left out to spoil, but rather either warmed or cooled to the preferred temperature and then eaten promptly. As to cold food, there is the added advantage of the chill actually numbing the pain. Very cold, even frozen, foods, may be helpful in this regard. Try icing beverages such as milk or juices. While ice cream, frozen yogurt, and sherbet are all good, the constant sweetness may become tiresome. Purees of savory foods may be chilled or even frozen into "Popsicles," or they may be frozen partially and stirred or blended to the consistency of soft ice cream. Small, inexpensive, hand-cranked iceless "ice cream freezers," such as that made by Donvier, can be kept in the freezer ready to use and are ideal for this purpose. Experiment with cold soups or by flavoring plain yogurt with savory flavors such as Worcestershire or soy sauce. Please note that with savory foods it is important that they be as fat- and grease-free as possible, as the coagulated fat would render them unpalatable. As the perception of salt is greatly reduced in cold foods, you may find that you prefer slightly oversalting your food when it is cold, providing you do not find that the salt causes irritation.

EASE IN SWALLOWING

In many cases you may find that holding your head at a certain angle may help reduce pain in swallowing. Try tilting your head forward or back or turning it to one side. Experiment. Rinsing your mouth with lukewarm salt water both immediately before and after eating also should help reduce your discomfort.

DRY MOUTH

If dry mouth is a problem for you, do as the raccoon does and moisten your food (this is the truth behind his "washing"). Add gravy, broth, or cream sauces to foods for moisture or take frequent sips of a beverage as you eat. Cold water with a touch of lemon is most refreshing. Carry a "sports bottle" of water with you and wet your mouth frequently. Between meals, sucking on hard candies (especially those that are sour) may help maintain a flow of saliva. Quench is a brand of chewing gum designed to stimulate saliva and quench thirst. If the problem of dry mouth persists, your doctor or dentist can prescribe artificial saliva drops.

SUGGESTED RECIPES
- Pimento cheese
- Salmon spread

- Liver pâté
- Hummus
- Egg drop soup
- Avgolemono
- Bean soup
- Quiche
- Chicken and dumplings
- Baked custard
- Cheesecake
- Sweetened sour cream
- Fruit gelatin
- Blender drinks

Renal Failure

Strides made in medicine have extended the average life span in the general population, thus bringing us new geriatric health problems that people who died at a younger age simply did not encounter. Similarly, the advances in HIV medicine have also far extended life expectancies. Renal problems were a later-stage development most people did not reach early in the epidemic, but which now occur with increasing frequency. With these problems come a new set of challenges unique to those experiencing renal failure.

Our kidneys are part of our body's mechanism for removing toxins, which they do by screening the blood. Toxins are substances that are poisonous by nature and also those things, such as sodium and potassium, which are necessary but toxic in excess. With renal (kidney) failure these various substances are not efficiently screened from the body and must be removed through dialysis—a mechanical screening of the blood. Simultaneously, to prevent their buildup it is necessary to restrict their intake. This may include restricting one or more of the following: calories, fluids, phosphorus, potassium, protein, or sodium. As you can see, these are all things elemental to a healthy diet. CAUTION: Do *not* use vitamin or other supplements except under the advice of your doctor or renal dietitian, as they may contain ingredients harmful to you.

Specific renal problems (and their severity) will determine what dietary modifications are appropriate. Typically, a person on dialysis will have her blood tested weekly to monitor and fine-tune both her treatment and diet. To meet these remarkably individualized needs, anyone with renal failure should work in concert with a dietitian who specializes in this field. With the renal dietitian as your primary source, the following suggestions are offered to help you work within the guidelines determined for your individual needs.

COPING STRATEGIES

FLUID RESTRICTION
Fluids frequently must be restricted for those on dialysis to prevent edema (swelling). A measured allowance of fluid is determined (usually the volume of your urine plus two cups) and all liquids consumed (in various forms, such as soup or ice) must be accounted for and subtracted from this allowance. A helpful technique for gauging the amount through the day is to have a clear pitcher filled with water equal to the daily allowance of fluid. Pour out equivalent amounts from the pitcher as fluids are consumed to gauge your remaining available fluid allowance.

THIRST
In times of fluid restriction, thirst is not an accurate guide to your body's need for fluid, though the problem of thirst still exists. Try the following:

- Many people find that ice is the most refreshing way to take their beverage allowance. Measure out that allotment and flavor the water with lemon juice or a touch of raspberry vinegar to make it more refreshing.

- Suck on sour hard candy or chew gum. Quench brand gum is specifically designed to quench thirst while *not* adding any electrolytes (potassium, sodium, or chloride).
- Rinse your mouth with very cold water, but do not swallow.
- Drink your beverage allowance ice cold, as cold beverages are more refreshing.
- Freeze slices of lemon to chew on.

POTASSIUM RESTRICTION

Potassium is best reduced in the diet by restricting those items listed below as "High Potassium." Please note that items (such as tomatoes) are not listed in all of their possible forms (juice, catsup, paste, sauce, et cetera) but that all forms would fall into generally the same category. Juices tend to be the concentrated essences of many things, so that they frequently will have the most potassium of any form of a given item.

Further reduction of potassium in vegetables can be achieved by peeling and cutting them into bite-sized pieces and soaking them in water to cover for two hours. They should then be drained, rinsed, and cooked in fresh water to cover. Potatoes should be cut into half-inch cubes, covered in ten times their volume of water, and allowed to soak overnight before draining, rinsing, and cooking.

High Potassium

Artichokes, avocados, bananas, beans, lentils and legumes (dried), collards, dates, figs, melons, molasses, oranges, potatoes (including sweet potatoes), processed anything, prunes, raisins, salt substitutes, spinach, tomatoes

Moderate Potassium

Apricots, corn, green peppers, kale, mushrooms, okra, peaches, pears, plums

Low Potassium

Apples, asparagus, beets, berries, broccoli, cabbage, carrots, celery, cherries, cranberries, cucumber, eggplant, grapefruit, grapes, green beans, lettuce, onions, tangerines, peas (not dried), pineapple, radishes, summer squash

PHOSPHORUS RESTRICTION

Phosphate binders are medical supplements that are by far the most effective method of dealing with excess phosphorus. They should be taken as prescribed by your doctor, in addition to your avoiding the foods listed below. If taking a phosphate binder causes constipation, ask your doctor for a stool softener

High Phosphorus

Artichokes, broccoli, chocolate, cola drinks, dairy products, dried beans, peas, lentils and legumes, egg yolks, greens, ham, lima beans, molasses, mushrooms, organ meats, nuts, peanut butter, shellfish, tofu, wheat

SODIUM RESTRICTION

Though many foods contain naturally occurring sodium, most salt that is consumed is added in cooking. Excess sodium causes fluid retention (edema or swelling) and thirst. In addition to salt added during cooking and at table, many foods are salt laden. To be avoided are:

- Monosodium glutamate (MSG), meat extracts and tenderizers
- Baking soda and baking powders (even "low sodium")
- Bottled sauces (catsup, chili, barbecue, mustard, soy, Worcestershire)
- Canned soups and bouillon
- Olives, pickles, sauerkraut
- Chocolate and cocoa
- Gravy and sauce mixes
- Canned vegetables (including baked beans)

- Lunch meats and hot dogs
- Cured meats (ham and bacon, corned beef, pastrami)
- Chinese food
- Processed foods (including cheeses and most frozen dinners)
- Chips, pretzels, and nuts
- "Softened" water

Please note that most salt substitutes contain potassium and are therefore not an acceptable substitute for renal-disease patients. To replace the "punch" sometimes lacking in a salt-restricted diet, try herbs and spices, dry vermouth, lemon juice, bitters (such as Angostura), or a range of flavored vinegars or oils, such as garlic and white wine vinegar or fennel-flavored oil.

PROTEIN

Protein from animal sources, being "complete proteins," leave fewer waste amino acids to be screened from the blood and therefore tax the kidneys least. Dairy products and eggs are those animal-source proteins which are most easily and completely utilized and absorbed by the body.

ADEQUATE CALORIC INTAKE

In a low-protein diet, if calories are not supplied by carbohydrates and fats, the body will steal from its stores of protein, jeopardizing lean body mass and producing toxic nitrogenous wastes (the same as if you'd eaten a high-protein, low-calorie diet). For this reason it is of great importance to maintain adequate caloric intake.

SPECIAL DIETARY PRODUCTS

Dietary Specialties
P.O. Box 227
Rochester, NY 14601
(716) 263-2787

Med-Diet Laboratories, Inc.
3050 Ranchview Lane
Plymouth, MN 55447
(612) 550-2020

Strategies for Weight Gain and Maintenance

As has been discussed in chapters 1 and 2 on wasting and special nutritional considerations, maintaining weight—and specifically your lean body mass—is of paramount importance. In fact, lean body mass has been shown a more reliable predictor of survival with HIV than T-cell counts. While safeguarding your weight is vitally important at all stages of HIV disease, different circumstances call for different strategies and responses. If lack of appetite remains a problem, you can consult your doctor about various appetite-stimulating medications such as Megace or Marinol. Growth hormone therapies are also being researched. Working with a reputable AIDS-knowledgeable dietitian or nutritionist can be of great help in creating and tailoring a diet that best suits your own life, circumstances, and medications.

FOR THE ASYMPTOMATIC HIV-POSITIVE INDIVIDUAL

Normal Weight

If your weight is in the normal range, it is best to optimize your health through diet simply by improving your basic eating habits and perhaps gaining a few pounds. This is not just a general nag to be a better person. For you to wait until involuntary weight loss occurs to make changes in your eating habits is like a diabetic waiting until he is in a coma before he changes his habits.

The place to start is to take stock of your diet and examine it for deficiencies. Perhaps you eat lots of vegetables but few fruits. A small problem, but there are nutritional advantages unique to both foods, so increasing your intake of fruits would help to improve your overall profile. Some people, especially when young, can seemingly survive on junk food and enthusiasm. The key word in that statement is *seemingly*. Many aspects of poor nutrition are not immediately apparent but can contribute to metabolic dysfunction later if allowed to persist.

Underweight

To be HIV-positive and underweight is to start out behind square one. Much of the challenge of guarding your health in the advance of HIV disease is guarding your weight. Building that, ideally in the form of lean body mass (muscle), is never so easy as when nausea, diarrhea, or other AIDS-related problems do not undermine the effort. Malnutrition is vastly easier to prevent than to reverse, and that prevention begins with building up a full complement of flesh. Being mindful of the basic necessary components of diet, all other extra calories are fair game here: fat calories, sugar calories, whichever foods you find enable you to increase your caloric intake. The target here is not to become "fat," but to carry a little extra weight. If you have it within you to become a body builder, you can carry a lot of extra muscle weight, though that is not required. What is important is to begin now rather than waiting for some reversal of health.

Overweight

Though a little extra fat weight may serve to counterbalance a slight involuntary weight loss, too much extra fat weight will not be of any great help, as lean body mass is always the vital element to preserving your good health. This is not the time, however, to "go on a diet" to lose weight; rather, it is a time to improve your eating and exercise habits and to allow a "natural correction" to occur slowly. Unless they do muscle-building exercises, most dieters in the general population lose lean body mass as well as fat when dieting. "Dieting" often results in slowed metabolism that frequently causes the weight to be regained as fat; hence the "yo-yo" syndrome of alternating weight loss and regain. For someone living with HIV that loss of lean body mass is a danger. And should weight loss continue beyond the target weight, malnutrition can occur. The concerns typically associated with excess weight (cholesterol, hypertension), unless extreme, are much less urgent than those of HIV.

Focus your eating on a wide-ranging, balanced intake of foods, gradually reducing your fat intake. Keep a food diary that includes "grazed" foods (which, if junk foods, are typically heavy on fat and short on quality nutrition). These records can help you identify where more nutritious, less fatty foods may be substituted in your diet. Consider beginning or increasing exercise. Don't expect change to occur overnight. The goal is to steadily move in a direction of increased lean body mass/decreased percentage body fat.

FOR SYMPTOMATIC INDIVIDUALS

If you are symptomatic, your body will be using more energy than normal in its efforts to fight infection. For every one degree of fever, your metabolic needs increase 7 percent. This means that even when experiencing a slight fever, ideally you would increase your food consumption 15–20 percent! Of course, this rarely happens. Few of us feel like eating at all when we have a fever. The particular symptoms you experience will determine which strategies to follow to gain or to maintain your weight, either when you are actively ill or between bouts of illness. For example: adding dry, powdered milk to your meat-loaf mixture would be a great nutritional add-on, but not if it induces lactose-intolerance diarrhea. A peanut-butter sandwich is good-quality, inexpensive protein, but not good for someone who has a great deal of trouble digesting fats. It is up to you to sort through the following suggestions and glean which are appropriate to your individual situation. Using them as guidelines, you may develop your own methods of enhancing your diet, tailored to your tastes and circumstances. Consulting with a reputable nutritionist would be helpful.

STRATEGIES TO GAIN AND MAINTAIN WEIGHT

THE WAY YOU EAT

Frequent Small Meals

Grazing is the enemy of people who diet to lose weight; it is your friend. It is much easier to take in more food over the course of a day if you do so in small, frequent snacks and meals, not three regimented sessions of eating. Example: a midmorning hard-boiled egg, afternoon peanut butter and crackers, bedtime cheese toast; that, alone, may *double* your day's protein intake, plus add substantial numbers of calories. Not overwhelming your system with great sudden quantities of food will also help avoid digestive upsets.

Atmosphere

Many things affect our appetites—even a dining room painted red has been proven to be more stimulating to the appetite than one painted blue. We tend to think our appetite is what it is, but in fact there are many things we can do to help enhance it. Consider which of the following might work for you.

Try eating in different places. Always eating in the kitchen or bedroom can have a deadening sameness which can kill appetite. Some cold winter night, get in a warm bath with a bowl of chili and think of the sleet outside. On a fine day, take a sandwich to the park or even to the backyard. Try putting a table just by the window, as in a restaurant, so that the passing scene, street or na-

ture, offers its own variation. There are many ways we can enhance our eating environment. Candles don't need to be tall, for-
mal tapers; even a small votive candle in an old jam jar will add
life to a table and a sense of occasion. Flowers may come from a
shop, or perhaps they may be found on an afternoon walk, growing wild. Or maybe not flowers, but a branch of interesting leaves
in a vase. Try putting a houseplant on the table (and changing it
frequently). Favorite music while eating can also add to enjoyment. In fact, reserving some favorite music to listen to only while
eating can help you look forward to mealtimes.

Presentation

The idea of variety extends to more than location. Variety in flavors, textures, and colors can all help stimulate appetite. Is Chinese food your favorite? Have Mexican food for a change. Always
eat chicken? Try pork. Even if you find you don't care for it much,
the chicken may look better to you when you come back to it. Or
maybe you'll find you like pork more than you remembered.
Color, too, can be an important variant. A meal of roast chicken,
scalloped potatoes, and braised celery would be a beige monot-
ony. Bright-green steamed broccoli and sautéed carrots would
give visual stimulation as well as a more complete range of nutrients. Chances are a meal with no red anywhere is missing not just
a top-note of color, but of flavor as well. Radishes, tomatoes,
strawberries, raspberries, red bell pepper—they all offer bright,
clear flavors as well as bright, clear colors, both of which help
stimulate the appetite. It is fascinating the degree to which a balance of colors in a meal is reflective of a balance of nutrients.

Community

The greatest variable, of course, is company. Eating with others
has been well proven to improve nutritional profiles through increased appetite and regularity of eating. This is true throughout
the general population, but is particularly true of those who are ill
or elderly. Too often the motivation to eat is simply not there.

Even those with pets are found to have better nutritional profiles; if we go into the kitchen to feed the cat, perhaps we eat something too. If we go to the store for dog food, we might pick up some supplies for our own dinner. For those who live alone or who are loners by nature, it may take some active efforts to cultivate dining companions. Company for every meal is not required, but you may discover that people are delighted to find that helping out may be as simple as sharing a meal. Accept invitations, even if you're feeling grumpy and out of sorts (and then try not to act as if you're feeling grumpy and out of sorts—maybe you'll be asked back). The pleasure of company is one of the greatest enhancements to eating. "Better is a dinner of herbs, where love is. . . ."

Food is one of the great pleasures of being alive. It is a communion of the spirit as well as the body. Almost all of us have treasured memories associated with food and almost all great celebrations have attendant feasting. If you have no appetite and cannot eat at a given time, do not yield to feelings of guilt or recrimination. Yes, it is better if you can eat; no, this is not a "moral" issue. Sadly, too many people who are suffering a temporary loss of appetite approach mealtimes with apprehension, feeling dread and avoidance—a state sometimes exacerbated by well-meaning caregivers who continually urge food. Surely nothing will kill an appetite more quickly or thoroughly than feelings of guilt, anxiety, and dread. Better to nurture your appetite back to vigor than to destroy the pleasure you can have in food.

WHAT YOU EAT

Fats

Nothing packs a caloric punch like fats. One gram of protein or carbohydrate equals 4 calories, 1 gram of fat equals 9! You can easily see how valuable fats become in efforts to gain weight. It is hard to maintain a high-calorie diet without a fairly substantial fat intake. There are, however, a couple of important points to keep in mind as you pile on the butter.

First, much of our feeling of "fullness" or satiety when eating comes not from the quantity of food we have eaten (as anyone who has tried to fill up on celery knows) but from our intake of fats, especially saturated fats. The absorption of saturated fats into the bloodstream quickly signals our brain to shut down the impulse of hunger. If we are trying to gain weight and are relying too heavily on fat calories, we can cease to be hungry before we've met our nutritional needs. A richly fat-marbled slice of beef may have more calories than a lean slice, but if that fat prevents us from eating as much as we would of a leaner cut, we may not get our full protein intake. If your appetite is slight, this is an important consideration. There are many ways to add caloric and nutritive value to foods; fat is but one. Do not rely on it entirely to increase your caloric intake, at the risk of diminished appetite.

The second consideration as you add fats to your diet is whether they will contribute to digestive problems, such as nausea or diarrhea. From time to time we all have difficulty digesting fats. Problems such as diarrhea, which may begin from completely unrelated causes, can be made worse by a diet high in fat. At such times it is much more important to correct the digestive problem by deleting fats from the diet, while taking whatever other measures are necessary.

Fluids

Though many health guidelines encourage us to drink more water, other beverages, such as fruit juices, will supply additional calories and other nutrients. Even "soft drinks" like colas and ginger ale (in their nondietetic forms) can help to add extra calories. Many "blender drinks" (see Part Four for recipes) can be virtual meals in themselves—or extra meals between meals. Try sugar and heavy cream in your coffee. If you like seltzer or iced tea, mix it by half with a favorite fruit juice. Sip on hot broth in the afternoon instead of a cup of tea. (Please note that while a clear soup is a good substitute for a beverage that does not contain much nutrition, it is a poor substitute for heartier "food" and it can be filling. Be careful of filling up on a thin soup at the expense of eating. See recipe for egg drop soup, page 163.)

Always Up the Ante

Are you having pie for dessert? How about a scoop of ice cream on top? Cereal for breakfast? Try adding some extra raisins or other dried fruit. Having a hamburger for lunch? Make it a cheeseburger. Get in the habit of looking at your meal-to-be and asking yourself, "How can I punch this up and make it more?"

SPECIFIC FOOD SUGGESTIONS

Following is a grab bag of suggestions for nutritious, calorie-laden foods, which may be used as add-ons to your regular diet:

Hard-Boiled Eggs

Eggs are the highest-quality protein available to the body and valuable nutrition packages besides; think of these as little protein/nutrition bullets. Since they keep well, make a dozen or two at a time and have them handy to snack on.

Snack Spreads

Lots of things handy to spread on crackers are packed with nutrition. Peanut butter is great. Canned liver pâté is very nutritious (and inexpensive). Cream cheese is excellent. Even many brands of crackers are astonishingly caloric—just read the labels.

Nuts

High-protein, high-calorie, good nutritious snack food.

Cheese

As with nuts, this is an excellent snack food and a complete protein. Cheeses come in great variety, so use this exploration to stimulate your appetite.

SUGGESTED RECIPES
- Pimento cheese
- Salmon spread
- Hummus
- Liver and onions
- Cheese casserole
- Meat loaf
- Vegetable casserole
- Cheesecake
- Peanut-butter cookies
- Blender drinks

Also see: Chapter 19, "Nutritional Enhancements for Everyday Foods."

ome 15

Accommodating Changes
in Taste Perception

Medications, changes in metabolism, or a combination of the two may contribute to altered taste perceptions that can undermine your enjoyment of food and thereby jeopardize your nutritional intake. This is an area that is quite subjective, so that some active participation in creative problem-solving will be the challenge if you are experiencing changes in taste.

In some cases, greater adherence to a good regimen of oral hygiene will help enormously. Not only is routine brushing and flossing necessary, but you may find that frequent rinsing, particularly before eating, helps a great deal. Brush with baking soda instead of toothpaste before meals. Toothpaste can leave an artificial taste in the mouth that creates taste alterations of its own.

Sometimes the taste changes experienced in food are not "bad," only "different." For many people this is the same thing. Flexibility (an identifying characteristic of long-term survivors) is important in regearing our expectations in these circumstances. Some people will only enjoy meat loaf if it is just the way they've always had it (probably the way their mom made it) and if it should have a Cheddar cheese topping instead of mozzarella, they consider it little short of the devil's work. These people are probably not going to do very well if they experience changes in taste perception. A little creativity and flexibility are what is called for here. Would a grind of pepper offset the "squashy" taste in a melon? Would some salt help the milkshake? Would lots of onion overwhelm the slight unpleasant taste in tunafish salad? Only you can judge.

To get around those preconceived notions which may disappoint you in foods you know well, try foods that are less familiar. There is a world of ethnic cooking available almost everywhere these days, and very few of us have eaten much of it. If you grew up with an Italian mama, go out for Chinese or Mexican food. If you've eaten Chinese food ever since you can remember, try Thai food for a change or Jewish cuisine. If you're a traditional southerner, explore northern Italian food. Not only can we dispense with many of our concepts of how food is "supposed" to taste by trying things that are genuinely foreign, but this pursuit can be one of the great pleasures of life (as opposed to sitting home complaining that the meat loaf just doesn't taste the same anymore). And *foreign* doesn't just mean "ethnic"; any food unfamiliar to us is foreign.

As you explore new foods, take notes about combinations of tastes and ingredients that intrigue and delight you. If you find that you like *tatzikia* (a traditional Greek sauce of yogurt, dill, cucumber, and garlic), might a pinch of dill help with an off taste in your morning yogurt? If, in some Middle Eastern restaurant or cookbook, you come across steamed pumpkin with ground lamb and yogurt, might you use these flavors at home with squash and ground beef and sour cream? By the way, this blending of international flavors and juxtapositions of ingredients is what is known as "fusion cooking" and is what is at the very forefront of cooking trends these days.

This all, of course, presupposes some basic cooking skills (or willingness to learn them), because no one can second-guess the subjective taste perceptions you may be experiencing. If someone else is cooking for you, you must make every effort to communicate how flavors taste bad or good to you; simply saying, "This tastes bad," offers no practical guidance. To say, "This meat tastes sour; this rice pudding tastes bitter," offers someone a clue as to how he might modify a dish to accommodate your tastes.

One of the more common taste changes of which people complain is that protein will sometimes seem to have a bitter or metallic taste. Since protein intake is of great concern for someone living with HIV, dealing with this problem is of great importance.

• As this perception is frequently most extreme in red meats, simply changing to poultry, seafood or fish may help.

• Some meats, such as pork or poultry, lend themselves well to fruit flavors (orange marmalade glazes, plum sauces, or sour cherry accompaniments, for example), which are very successful at offsetting bitter or metallic tastes. Cheese eaten with fruit will also have this same counterbalancing effect.

• Marinades and condiments such as chutneys can also help manipulate flavors.

• Try eating meats (or any protein that may have a bitter or metallic taste) cold. A hearty sandwich is a good solution here.

• Meat in small pieces added to soups or casseroles is another way to minimize its contribution to the overall taste of a dish and still maintain protein intake.

• Eating with plastic utensils may be found to help. If you notice an improvement from switching to plastic utensils, look around flea markets or yard sales for some odd pieces of inexpensive silver-plated flatware (whose silver is not all worn off). Silver has much less of a metallic taste than steel and for under ten dollars you might find that you can greatly enhance your eating enjoyment.

• Consider protein sources other than meats, such as eggs, beans and legumes, and dairy products.

Whether we maintain or lose the delight we take in food is an important quality-of-life indicator. In addition to taste changes wrought by medications or metabolic changes, depression can alter perceptions of food, as of all of life. Not uncommonly, food will taste bland and uninteresting to people who are finding life bland and uninteresting. Since the joy we take in eating is one of the surest factors in determining our involvement with food and therefore our nutritional profiles, psychological factors must be considered in any assessment determining lack of food intake. Psychological counseling and medications must be considered as valid nutritional therapies for those who have lost interest in eating.

SUGGESTED RECIPES
- Orange glazed chicken
- Ginger sherry pork chops
- Seasonal chutneys
- Flavored vinegars and oils

Nutritional Supplements and Total Parenteral Nutrition (TPN)

LIQUID FOOD SUPPLEMENTS

Maintaining the function of your gut so that it does not atrophy from lack of use will be of great importance to you if you have difficulty eating for any extended time. Specially formulated canned supplements, such as Ensure, are now widely available and are excellent products. They provide complete nutrition in a formulation designed for optimal absorption and can help you to sustain gut function when standard foods are not tolerated. They can also be used to supplement nutritional intake if your normal diet is reduced for any reason.

Some supplements, such as Advera, are designed especially to meet the needs of people living with AIDS. Two great drawbacks to these are their taste and their high cost. They tend to have a "canned" flavor and a lingering aftertaste due to certain nutritionally potent components such as fish oil. Many little tricks, such as combining them in a blender with fresh fruit, will help improve their palatability. Most manufacturers provide recipe booklets giving a variety of ways to use and augment their products. (Ross Laboratories, makers of Advera and Ensure (800) 544-7495; Mead Johnson, makers of Lipisorb, Boost, and Sustacal (800)

247-7893, and Clintec, maker of Nutren, (800) 422-2752.) In almost all cases people seem to find the chocolate-flavored products most agreeable. You can enhance these liquid supplements further by adding a little cocoa powder or instant chocolate drink mix. Peppermint extract or instant coffee may also help.

Some health-insurance providers, recognizing that good nutrition provides a cost/value by helping to prevent a worsening of health problems, have begun to underwrite the cost of food supplements. This varies by state, so check with your doctor to see if he or she is able to prescribe it for you under some reimbursement plan.

Perhaps the greatest single advantage of these food supplements is that they provide a balanced nutritional complement without the use of dairy products. This obviates the potential problem of lactose intolerance. However, the considerable expense of these products makes the use of fortified milk well worth considering as a supplement if lactose intolerance is not a problem or if it can be managed through the use of lactase supplements, such as Lactaid or Dairy Ease. (For a more thorough discussion of lactose intolerance, see page 78.) **One cup of skim milk fortified with ¼ cup of powdered milk supplies *more* protein than one cup of standard canned nutritional food supplement and as much as one cup of high-energy supplement!** Instant-meal products, such as Carnation Instant Breakfast, can supply an even greater and wider complement of nutrients (when mixed with milk). If lactose intolerance is not a problem for you, or if you can manage the problem with a lactase supplement, this is by far your best value.

A final word about food supplements: they are supplements, not substitutes. There is no substitute for "real" food with its complex balance of micronutrients and trace elements. No supplement, however valuable, can ever adequately supply these subtle components of a healthy diet.

ENTERAL NUTRITION OR TUBE FEEDING

If problems with food intake are due to difficulties in the upper digestive tract (such as debilitating mouth and throat soreness) or to chronic debilitating nausea, your doctor may prescribe enteral nutrition or "tube feeding." This allows natural absorption/digestion to continue, thereby maintaining gut function and intestinal integrity. Liquid food supplements are given either via a nasal tube entry into the stomach or, for more extended periods, through a tube called a "PEG" (for Percutaneous Endoscopic Gastrostomy tube) into the side, connecting to the stomach.

PARENTERAL NUTRITION OR INTRAVENOUS FEEDING

In times of extreme inability to eat or lack of gut function, intravenous feeding or peripheral parenteral nutrition (PPN), either partial or total, can supply nutrients when no other dietary intake is possible. Partial parenteral nutrition can supplement and bolster your diet when only extremely limited food intake is possible (for whatever reason), and total parenteral nutrition (TPN) serves to provide complete nutritional support. This is administered in hospital settings or by home infusion companies whose business it is to instruct in the use and to oversee the home dispensing of their product. In strategies for preventing life-threatening weight loss and starvation, this technique can be a modern miracle.

Though it is possible to provide complete nutritional support with TPN, to prevent atrophy of the gut it is important to maintain whatever oral or enteral food intake is possible. Unfortunately, many people have come to look upon use of parenteral nutrition as a failure of body function and therefore evidence of inevitable and irreversible decline. As different stages of HIV disease call for different strategies and responses, parenteral nutrition can be one of the most effective tools for both the short- and long-term assurance of adequate sustenance.

Far from being a step down into irreversible dependence, parenteral nutrition can often provide a bridge through a course of illness, whereby additional ground is not lost in the form of body mass. Just eight months ago a friend of mine began partial parenteral nutrition during a lengthy hospital stay when food intake became problematic. After several months of relying on this supplementation, he recovered sufficient health not only to resume normal eating, but also to travel and vacation here and abroad. Such a recovery would have been virtually impossible had his weight loss not been checked and adequate nutrition maintained.

Parenteral nutrition requires the installation of a "port," a relatively permanent IV entry into the body through which blood may also be drawn and drugs administered. Installation is a relatively minor surgical procedure. (The IV may also be referred to as a "Hickman" or a "PICC" line, for "peripherally inserted central catheter"). A port dramatically reduces the number of times someone must be subjected to needle sticks. Infection can occur at these sites, so compliance with hygiene routines is very important.

Dramatic involuntary weight loss is of grave concern and all necessary measures should be taken, as needed, to avert it. If you feel it may be appropriate in your circumstances, discuss the matter with your doctor. You may also be able to receive detailed information from a home infusion company in your area. If you cannot locate one in your telephone directory, try asking for a referral from your hospital, local health department, or AIDS service organization.

SUGGESTED RECIPES

See pages 197–200 for techniques and recipes to make liquid supplements more palatable.

PART FOUR

Cooking Techniques and Recipes

Basic Principles of Cooking Protein

The importance of adequate protein intake for someone living with HIV justifies this subject's having its own chapter, the essence of which can be stated in a single sentence: **High heat toughens protein.**

This is true of all proteins: eggs, meats, cheeses, you name it.* Eggs fried at a high heat might just as well be used to sole shoes. Meat cooked at a high temperature becomes tough and stringy. Cheese grated into a soup that is at a rolling boil turns mealy and rubbery and never melts. Protein, in all of its forms, responds badly when subjected to high heat.

Do not worry that this is a matter of undercooking. Even a tough cut of meat like pot roast becomes meltingly tender, and flavorful, when cooked at a gentle heat for a long period of time. The same degree of doneness (i.e., internal temperature) will ultimately be reached, but the results are far from the same. Resist the temptation to crank up the heat when you're cooking and you will be rewarded with food that is more flavorful, more nutritious, and more tender.

---

* For an exhaustive examination of this subject, see Adelle Davis's *Let's Cook It Right,* published by NAL-Dutton, New York, 1988.

Selection, Storage, and Cooking of Vegetables and Fruits

There are many wonderful and elaborate recipes for fruit and vegetable dishes of every sort, but for our day-to-day purposes, simple preparations of seasonal, prime vegetables serve most of our needs. Here are the basic methods of selection, storage, and preparation, with an eye toward nutrition, taste, and visual appeal.

SELECTION

In fruits and vegetables, as with the human face, genuine goodness is often reflected in a humble and homely beauty. Anyone who has sampled a variety of apples knows this. Perfect form and unblemished surface are frequently reflective of a hothouse origin and not the variable and natural growth of produce shaped and flavored by the sun and soil.

When choosing vegetables, look, instead, for those whose color and form suggest a full, young ripeness when harvested. This does not mean excessive size or a bloated fullness, but rather a "filling out" of their natural size. For example, a tomato with high shoulders near the stem straining to ridges down its sides is apt to be tasteless and pithy. Better one that is gently rounded in its form.

A relative heaviness of any individual vegetable or piece of fruit indicates juiciness (from the added weight of the water content). This is especially noticeable in fruits such as grapefruit. The skin should be thin and you should be able to feel the slightly yielding flesh beneath it, indicating ripeness. Obviously this quality and degree of "firm yielding" will vary tremendously depending on whether a peach or a squash is being selected, but in all cases there should be no "dry, hollow" feeling, as though the piece were stuffed with tightly packed sawdust. The color should be vivid, indicating sufficient exposure to sunlight (on whose development nutritiously valuable phytochemicals depend). The old test of fragrance is enormously valuable if the fruits and vegetables have not been highly refrigerated, but not only does chill significantly reduce the volatility of fragrance oils—in many cases it actually destroys enzymes which actively contribute to a vegetable's distinct flavor. This is why a refrigerated tomato, even if brought back to room temperature, does not have the same fullness of flavor as one that has never been chilled. If you are lucky enough to buy your fruits and vegetables from a true farm stand or farmers' market, you'll notice that tomatoes have a tantalizing, lingering acrid fragrance, cantaloupes smell of melon and not of old squash, and indeed, each fruit and vegetable has a unique and appealing smell of its own.

ORGANIC PRODUCE

There is scant evidence that organically grown produce is significantly more nutritious than that grown by conventional methods. Many times, due to its greater expense, it does not sell as rapidly, compromising its freshness and negatively counterbalancing any slight nutritional advantage it may have begun with. Of more serious concern is that much organic produce is fertilized with natural compost fertilizers, which are usually composed with raw manure. This can lead to serious food safety concerns, as many pathogenic agents are transferred fecally. For produce that can be washed, peeled, and cooked, this problem is lessened, but vegetables such as lettuce which are eaten raw cannot be made safe and should not be eaten.

STORAGE

Fruits and vegetables are at their utmost prime on the vine, stalk, or tree. Some, such as corn, begin to deteriorate from the moment they are picked, so that devotees who grow their own will bring cooking water to a boil before heading out to pick the ears they intend to serve. In July and August every rural highway has hand-lettered signs announcing "local corn." Others, such as pineapples, will never increase their sugar content after harvest. Since this is largely the measure of a fruit's flavor, if picked early they are held in a state of unripeness. Some produce, like pears or tomatoes, will continue to ripen, though never to the degree of perfection as if left on the branch where they grew. Having selected the best produce you can obtain, it is important to keep it at its peak of freshness, both for reasons of flavor and of nutrition.

First, let's make a distinction which may seem technical but which has practical applications: Anything that is the seed and ovary system of a plant is a fruit; thus, tomatoes, corn, squashes, beans, and green peppers are all actually fruits. Foods from other parts of the plant are vegetables; thus celery, potatoes, broccoli, and lettuce are all vegetables. As we all know, plants "breathe in" carbon dioxide and expel oxygen, just as we do the reverse. Lesser known is that *fruits* need oxygen, or they wither and die. You might think of an old-fashioned ceramic fruit bowl that has many perforations to allow air passage and circulation (just like a basket). To keep your fruits (again, those "vegetables" such as cucumbers or peas) wrapped in the plastic bags or shrink-wrapped containers from the grocery store is to cause them needless loss of both nutrients and flavor. It is true that plastic will prevent moisture loss, but the same thing will be accomplished by a damp towel or the natural humidity of a vegetable crisper compartment of a refrigerator.

If you want to bring fruits to greater ripeness, the old "banana in a brown paper bag" is an excellent technique, providing that you punch a number of holes in the bag to allow some flow of oxygen. The reason for this is that most fruits give off ethylene gas, a natural agent that stimulates ripening. The denser the immediate environment is with this gas, the more quickly most fruits ripen; therefore it is necessary to contain it. Some fruits produce the gas in abundance (bananas are virtual factories of ethylene gas) and you may harness it from one to encourage ripening in another. In other words, if you put a banana in a perforated brown paper bag with a tomato, it will hasten the ripening of the tomato.

Most people who bring home a slightly wilted bunch of flowers know exactly what to do: give the stems a fresh cut and place them upright in lukewarm water. For some reason these same people will cook withered broccoli or throw out slightly limp celery, which, more often than not, just needs a little drink of water to be restored to perfect freshness. This is true for any cut-stem vegetable, such as asparagus or parsley, which also may be kept fresh for much longer periods if kept in water. Other things can be restored to crispness by a soak in cold water. Remarkably flaccid lettuce can be torn for salad and covered with ice water and returned to crispness, as can carrots. Please note that it is preferable to keep vegetables fresh in the first place, as this soaking can leach out water-soluble vitamins. However, if the alternatives are no lettuce, wilted lettuce, or "restored" lettuce, by all means opt for the last.

All produce should, of course, be thoroughly washed to remove any lingering pesticide or trace of fertilizer.

COOKING

For conversational ease while discussing cooking methods, I use the term *vegetables* in the common use of the word and not in the technical sense of vegetables versus fruits. By now we all know that cooking vegetables in great quantities of water until they are little better than mush destroys virtually all of their nutritional value. However, the modern notion of "Less is more" in cooking vegetables cannot be extended indefinitely. Yes, vegetables retain more of their nutritional value if cooked only lightly so as to retain a degree of their natural body or "crunch." No, all cooking is not bad. In fact, cooking makes many nutritional components of vegetable and other foods more bioavailable to you. Let's examine some simple methods of cooking vegetables.

Boiling

Boiling is probably the least nutritionally advantageous method of cooking vegetables, as many water-soluble compounds are lost in the process. True, you can retrieve the compounds by using these "vegetable waters" as the bases for soups, or simply by drinking them, but almost no one ever does this to the degree that they are produced if this is your primary manner of cooking vegetables. If boiled is the only way you like vegetables, try cooking them in as little briskly boiling water as possible for as brief a time as you can. In the moments between cooking and serving them, remove the vegetables from the pan and, while keeping them warm, reduce the liquid down to a few tablespoons by boiling it rapidly. Serve this "liquor" over the vegetables and you will thus retain as much of the water-soluble vitamins as possible. Or, if it is more convenient than keeping them warm during the reducing process, simply stir the vegetables back in during the last few minutes of reducing the liquid. Just be sure neither to burn them nor overcook them (having wisely removed them from the water underdone in anticipation of this later re-heating/cooking).

Steaming

Steaming is a much better technique for retaining nutrients in vegetables, though significant vitamin loss does still occur—just look at the water left in the pan after you've steamed broccoli. The same suggestions for reusing these "vegetable waters" apply, else those vitamins simply go down the drain. The advantage here is that the much smaller quantity of liquid left from steaming makes it easier to incorporate these waters into other foods, and thereby into your diet.

Utensils for steaming vary widely and some are much more efficient to use, and to clean, than others. Very common is a steaming basket composed of a perforated disk on short legs, ringed by overlapping perforated petals that open or narrow to fit into a variety of pots and pans. Though this object accomplishes the steaming perfectly well, it is difficult to keep completely clean, as its recesses trap foods which are hard to remove even with thorough washing. These devices also tend to be fragile and to shed their petals, necessitating their frequent replacement and making their slight expense a false economy.

Perhaps the easiest steamer to use and clean is one made like a double boiler with perforations in the bottom and sides of the insert. This is also easier and safer to handle when removing the vegetables from the hot pan in which they have cooked. Such an arrangement may be improvised with a colander or strainer set over a pan with a scant amount of water in the bottom and as close-fitting a lid as possible.

Microwaving

Microwave cooking of vegetables is an excellent method from a standpoint of nutrition, flavor, and color. No additional water is required after washing, so that vitamin loss is kept to an absolute minimum. Even if vegetables are shaken virtually completely dry, there is still plenty of moisture within the vegetable to effect the cooking process that follows.

Vegetables should be cut into regular, bite-sized pieces and placed in a nonmetal bowl. Cover this with plastic wrap and cook the vegetables until they are just underdone (the time will depend on amount being cooked and wattage of the microwave oven). Then allow them to sit for a minute or two to complete their cooking process. Special microwave cookware is available for this purpose. As there is almost no residual liquid left from cooking vegetables this way, water-soluble vitamins are retained to the greatest degree possible. Quick and easy, microwaving vegetables is a method to be highly recommended.

Sautéeing and Stir-Frying

These techniques are Western and Eastern variations on the same theme and this method of cooking vegetables is highly recommended. In addition to being waterless and therefore retaining water-soluble vitamins, colors remain bright and the slight browning adds savor. It has two further great advantages.

First, in other methods of cooking vegetables, moisture, even from steam, remains on the surface. When butter is applied, much of it slides off, like the proverbial water off a duck's back. The same vegetable gently sautéed in the same butter has its surface permeated as the steam is constantly driven off. The vegetables are bathed in the cooking fat (butter or oil) as they cook, which gives them not only a delicious flavor but also valuable added calories.

Second, it is easy to add a little flavoring as you cook vegetables this way and dramatically change the nature of the dish—an important consideration in the throes of winter when all too often broccoli seems to be the only fresh vegetable to be had for weeks on end. A splash of soy sauce in the sauté will give a completely different flavor. Or garlic might be added to the oil. With minimal effort you can easily effect many changes.

My favorite vegetable dish is most easily achieved with this method of cooking: a vegetable medley. It is extremely nutritious in its variety, it can be assembled from whatever vegetables are seasonally available, and it is the most economical way to use up odds and ends of vegetables. And it looks and tastes great! Look for a variety of colors: The odd stalk of broccoli too little for a single serving, the loose carrot in the vegetable drawer; add to these a summer squash and some red bell pepper and you have a fine medley. Chop vegetables into bite-sized pieces and add them to the skillet (with butter or oil) one at a time, beginning with those needing the longest cooking times (generally the hardest). You might begin with some sliced carrot and some cauliflower; after a few moments add some red bell pepper and zucchini; toward the end add some green peas or asparagus. Leftover, previously cooked vegetables can be added at the end just long enough to heat through.

For a full meal, cooked meat can be added and the whole stir-fry served over rice. If there is anything left, add some broth and call it vegetable soup. As you see, this method can be developed in many directions.

A wide-ranging diet is our greatest assurance of adequate and balanced nutrition. Nowhere is that more true than in our consumption of vegetables. There is no one perfect vegetable that meets all of our needs, no matter how much of it we eat. To satisfy the vast array of our complex biochemical needs, a wide variety of fruits and vegetables is essential.

Nutritional Enhancements for Everyday Foods

A wide-ranging, balanced diet is, without question, the best route to good nutrition. Just as vitamin tablets are supplements, not substitutes for a good diet, no add-ons will ever make up for sporadic, unbalanced eating habits. Nutritional enhancements are just that: enhancements. Do not be misled into thinking that shoveling wheat germ onto your morning cereal, feasting on hot dogs, and never seeing a vegetable will all balance itself out. All sound diet must be predicated on balance and proportion (see Chapter 2, "Basic Nutrition"). With that said, the following are ways to add various nutrients (and especially protein) into foods you already eat.

NONINSTANT POWDERED MILK

For those who have no lactose-intolerance problem, noninstant powdered milk is a great nutritional boost that may be incorporated into an amazing array of foods. ("Instant" powdered milk does not offer nearly the equal nutritional advantage.) Even the milk you drink may be fortified to substantially boost its protein. In fact, one cup of skim milk fortified with ¼ cup powdered milk has more protein than a small chicken breast! Since powdered milk is nonfat, its addition does not make the foods it is added to more filling—a particular advantage if early satiety is a problem. Meat loaf, oatmeal, casseroles, baked goods, sauces, and scrambled eggs are all places where you might sneak in a little powdered milk.

WHEAT GERM

Wheat germ is the nutritional essence of wheat. Ounce for ounce it has nearly three times the protein of regular unbleached flour, and is an excellent source of B vitamins and other nutrients besides. Its nutty crunch is a welcome addition to many foods: yogurt, ice cream, fresh fruit, and breakfast cereal. It, too, can be snuck in many places unnoticed, such as meat loaf, casseroles, and baked goods.

HARD-BOILED EGGS

Eggs are the highest-quality and most readily digested protein. In addition to having them as snacks just as they are, you may slice and add them to a sandwich, chop and sprinkle them onto any variety of salad, many soups and, yes, add them to that damn meat loaf.

DRIED FRUITS AND NUTS

Nuts and dried fruits are calorie- and nutrition-dense foods that balance areas of the diet which otherwise may be lacking. Most granolas contain some of both, but that is no reason you can't add more or add them to other cereals. Salads, yogurt, ice cream, are all likely places to add these as well as to desserts such as rice pudding or cheesecake.

BACON

Bacon (wonderful bacon!) can be happily added to many sandwiches (ever try peanut butter and bacon?), or crumbled onto vegetables, salads, and casseroles for extra protein and calories.

GELATIN

Though gelatin is that rare exception, an incomplete animal-source protein, it may still be used to increase protein in foods with the understanding that it must be balanced with complementary proteins from other sources in the diet. Even when its congealing property is not desired, gelatin can still be incorporated to advantage. For example, a bouillon cube dissolved in hot water never quite tastes like chicken soup but rather like chicken "tea" because it lacks the natural gelatins that give soups a substance aside from mere strength of flavor. Introducing gelatin will give the liquid a "body" that will make it more like soup while adding valuable protein. This may be done with any soup, stew, or sauce. For each cup of liquid, simply soften 1 Tbs. (1 envelope) of gelatin in 1/4 cup of cool liquid for about 5 minutes; then stir into your soup. That's all.

OATMEAL

Oats are quite a nutritious grain and may be substituted for bread crumbs in many recipes. (Do I hear a meat loaf calling?) It can also be whirled in a blender to make oat flour, which may be used to nutritional advantage instead of regular flour when dredging foods or used half and half with regular flour in many baked goods.

20

Handy Foods: When You're Too Tired or Sick to Cook

At times when we are too exhausted to prepare food for ourselves, it is not only important to keep eating, it is perhaps more important than when we are well. As our immune systems wage war against opportunistic infections, our metabolic needs increase. The listlessness we may feel has to do in part with the body's shutting down "unnecessary operations," as in a state of siege. Nutrition is the fuel that keeps that battle going.

CONVENIENT FOODS

Here is where convenience foods offer us their greatest value. Do not, however, misinterpret "convenience" to mean "junk" foods. With a little care it is perfectly possible to eat intelligently and well with minimal effort. To do this a little preplanning is in order.

A well-stocked pantry is your first ally here. Many canned goods and "instant" products will keep almost indefinitely and provide a hearty meal in very short order with minimal effort. Remember all of those recipes from the 1950s that began with "Take a can of Cream of Mushroom soup . . ."? Use them! It is amazing how good they can be if given a little freshening up. Sometimes all that is needed is a little grind of fresh pepper, an added pinch of an herb, or a splash of sherry. Since "freshness" is usually what is missing in the taste of such foods, a small chop of onion or celery or bell pepper might offset a "canned" flavor and brighten the taste (see "Easy Seasonings," page 158). Example: A box of instant scalloped potatoes and a can of salmon might stay on the shelf for a year waiting for that cold, rainy night when you don't feel like going out. Combined, they would make a hearty and nutritious casserole. With a little diced celery and onion added it would make an even better casserole. Or try heating a can of unreconstituted cream soup and adding some chopped hard-boiled egg. Just before serving, flavor with a touch of dry sherry and serve over toast for a comforting supper. Or instead of hard-boiled egg, add leftover or canned chicken or tuna or bacon and serve over instant rice. At minimal effort you have supplied your body with fuel and protein. Consider punching up the nutritional component of either of these by adding some noninstant powdered milk (which will also keep on the shelf indefinitely).

Newer to the market are irradiated foods. You may have noticed cartons of milk that need no refrigeration until opened; this is because irradiation has rendered the contents sterile. As long as the individual package is not compromised, it will remain safe to eat. More and more foods are becoming available conserved in this manner: beef stew, vegetable dishes, complete meals. IRRADIATION IS A PERFECTLY SAFE WAY TO PRESERVE FOOD. In fact, its sterility is a great safeguard against food poisoning. No residual radiation contaminates the food (as is commonly feared). Irradiated food products need no refrigeration, are ready to eat just by heating them, and will keep until the stars go out. Their variety can allow greater selection to your "on-hand" stockpile of comestibles.

Frozen foods strike a happy balance between convenience, length of conservation, and freshness of final product. The "TV dinners" of old have come a long way. Vegetable side dishes, entrees, complete meals, specialty sandwiches, pastries, and desserts are all available. Also increasingly available are products

CONVENIENT ITEMS FOR A
WELL-STOCKED PANTRY

Canned meats
Ham, corned beef, chili, beef stew

Canned fish
Tuna, salmon, sardines

Grains and cereals
Pastas, converted rice, oatmeal, grits, cream of wheat, crackers, pretzels, breakfast cereals, ramen noodles

Dried beans and legumes
Split peas, black beans, kidney beans, lentils
Canned fruits
Canned vegetables
Canned soups
Peanut butter
Nuts, seeds, dried fruits
Noninstant powdered milk

designed not as ends in themselves but as assists to cooking. Mixtures of vegetables intended as the base for a soup or a stir-fry are an example. Consider combining unreconstituted Cream of Mushroom soup, leftover or canned chicken meat, some frozen mixed vegetables, and frozen pie dough for a chicken pot pie better than many moms used to make. Preparation time: ten minutes.

Of course you can freeze foods you make yourself for future use, both finished product and streamlined ingredient. If you're making a casserole, rather than make a large one and live on reheated leftovers, divide it and freeze what you're not going to eat at a single meal. Make an extra-large batch and freeze several for future meals. The effort to make a larger batch of any given dish is much less than making a smaller batch several times.

When you make something that doesn't lend itself to freezing for future meals, you can still save effort by making a large batch; the trick is not to get tired of eating the same food as leftovers seemingly forever. If you make a large batch of tuna salad, have it with lettuce and fruit at one meal, as a sandwich at another and as a tuna melt for yet a third.

Keep a stock of handy ingredients available frozen in small quantities. Cooked hamburger meat can easily be dropped into a (canned) vegetable soup to make a hearty stew or added to minute rice with some vegetables for an ersatz but delicious stir-fry (my own mother called this "American fried rice"). Cooked chicken meat may be made into pot pies, soups, chicken and dumplings, salad, casseroles, stir-frys. Cooked chicken is such an extremely versatile ingredient that it is well worth keeping on hand. Whenever you boil or roast a chicken, consider making extra just for this purpose.

STICK-IN-YOUR-FACE FOODS

When you are really too tired or ill to do any meal preparation at all, there are still nutritious foods that are ready to eat as is. Review your resources. Is there a meals-delivery service organization in your area? Many are specifically geared to people living with HIV, delivering hot ready-to-eat meals. Perhaps this is a time to stretch your budget to include some takeout or delivered food. Many Chinese restaurants have menus of least expense. Have friends or family members or co-workers offered to help out? Tell them now would be a good time. It is not rare that many people who would like to help are thwarted in their kindness by not knowing how or when they might be of service. Making an extra portion of a dinner that they are already preparing may be one of the simplest and most effective ways for them to share (and for you to accept) their love for you.

Many foods we think of as snack foods are really quite nutritious. However, general nutrition is not the point here. If our health is such that we don't feel like doing any food preparation whatsoever, chances are that our food intake is down too. At these times it is important that we prioritize our eating and make sure of getting those most important nutrients: protein and calories. For that reason fruit (excellent for purposes of *general* nutrition) would not be a wise choice at this time, for it supplies little of either. Snack cracker foods such as cheese, peanut butter, sardines, hummus, pâtés, salmon spreads, or cream cheese are all excellent for these dual purposes. The latter may be flavored with most any of the easy seasonings (listed on page 158) for variety. Hard-boiled eggs, which may be deviled or eaten plain, are also a dependable standby. (A calorie-adding compromise is to have them with a little mayonnaise.)

Finally, food supplements, such as Advera, can help augment and bolster diet during times when any effort beyond actual eating is apt to prove too taxing.

COOKING TECHNIQUES

If you're not feeling up to par, just about any kitchen chore is easier done while sitting rather than standing. Consider a high kitchen stool for countertop work (even washing dishes) or working at a low table, seated. Be sure to assemble all of your work ingredients first, so that you don't have to get up a number of times.

Slow Cookers

Slow cookers, such as Crock-Pots, are an excellent and safe method of setting up dinner early in the day (even as you leave for work in the morning) and, without further effort, having dinner waiting for you, complete, later in the evening. These cookers reach a temperature just above that required for safety and maintain that temperature over an extended time—an ideal way in which to cook any protein and especially appropriate for less tender cuts of meat (which can be among the most flavorful). A surprisingly wide variety of foods lend themselves to being cooked this way. Refer to the manual that will come with the appliance, as different capacities and wattages will cause individual recipes to vary.

Clay-pot Cooking

Famous for their delicious results in roasting poultry (but excellent for many other things besides) are clay cookers such as the Romertopf and Schlemmertopf cookers. These are covered baking dishes made of an especially porous clay that is soaked in water before being used. As the baking progresses, the moisture held by the clay assures that what is being roasted does not dry out. Toward the end of cooking all the moisture is evaporated and the food being cooked browns beautifully.

Fish and meats are excellent when prepared this way. Two words of advice: Buy the largest model clay pot that you think you may use. If a clay pot becomes crowded, things tend to stick to the walls and are difficult to manage. Also, though these cookers can be the devil to clean if you try to do so immediately after roasting, washing is simplicity itself if you will soak the cooker overnight. This will also eliminate the need for vigorous scrubbing, which will grind away at the surface and eventually block the pores of the clay. These cookers come with instruction/recipe booklets that will familiarize you with the various basic technique of using the model you select.

Clay-pot Roast Chicken

Simply "water the cooker" by letting it soak for ten to fifteen minutes (as per the manufacturer's instructions), put in the chicken (and any optional vegetables), cover, put in a cold oven, turn on the heat, and, in a little over an hour, come back to a perfectly roasted chicken. You may incorporate any seasonings or flavorings such as bay leaves or vermouth, which will delicately infuse the flavor of the dish.

Microwave Cooking

Microwave ovens are ideal not only for the heating and reheating of foods that have already been cooked, but also for the actual cooking of a wide variety of foods. From making the best oatmeal to steaming vegetables with minimal vitamin loss, there are many advantages to streamlined microwave cooking that should not be overlooked. Disappointments usually come from expecting microwave cookery to do everything the same as conventional methods. Though many proteins (such as meats) are toughened in microwave cooking and are therefore not likely candidates for this method, fish, which is gently and lightly cooked, can be wonderful when done this way. As with steaming vegetables, simply covering the fish with plastic wrap will contain enough moisture that the combination of steaming and microwaving will cook most fish in a matter of moments and with a delicacy lost by many other methods. More homely but equally nutritious meals can be put together quickly from a well-stocked pantry. Microwave ovens do a wonderful job of baking potatoes. When one is almost done, try topping it with a can of chili con carne and perhaps a grating of Cheddar cheese for an extra-easy high-protein meal. (Also see Microwave Cooking re: "Food Safety," page 58.)

Blender Drinks

Blender drinks can be a nutritional mainstay if composed with an eye to protein and calories. To this end, dairy products should be prime ingredients. Ice cream, yogurt, cottage cheese, and milk powders can all boost protein and calories *if* lactose is not a problem (see "Lactose Intolerance," page 78). If you have problems digesting dairy products that are not corrected by using a lactase supplement such as Lactaid, soy or rice-milk substitutes may be used. Because of the very real danger of salmonella food poisoning, raw eggs should be scrupulously avoided in any blender drink. Flavorings can range from peanut butter to fresh or frozen fruits and berries to the many exotic flavoring syrups (from passion fruit to anise). Variety of tastes is rarely a problem if you develop an enthusiasm for these handy meal/drinks. For a couple of recipes to get you started, see page 195.

Food Processors and Hand Blenders

Food processors and hand blenders serve to ease the part of food preparation that is frequently the most dreary and time consuming. (If they would only wash dishes after a meal, they would be perfect!) Get hold of one, master its many uses, and it will repay you well by streamlining your efforts in the kitchen.

Also see "Easy Seasonings," page 158.

Budget Eating without Nutritional Sacrifice

There are two basic rules of eating well even on the strictest budget and they both presuppose a rudimentary knowledge of cooking.

1. Use everything up. Don't throw anything away that can be used. Stalks from broccoli can be pureed in a blender with some milk (or half-and-half) and a little thickener (instant or leftover mashed potatoes or flour) and made into broccoli soup. Though soups are a likely candidate for almost any leftover, many other things offer themselves as vehicles. The meat from a chicken leg and a small portion of peas might be stir-fried with some rice, splashed with a little soy sauce, and become a fine lunch. Even leftover scrambled eggs can be added to this type of fried rice. Or the same chicken and peas could be folded into an omelet. Or put into a small baking dish, a little (leftover?) gravy added, and the whole thing topped off with biscuit dough and baked. The point is never, ever to throw anything away—no matter how little—that has valid food/nutrition potential. Even the bones after you've finished a roast chicken can be simmered slowly to make the base for a wonderful homemade chicken soup. Just add a little rice. (Have

any left from that chicken dinner? Did you think to make a little extra just for this purpose?) Or chicken vegetable. (You did have vegetables with that chicken dinner, didn't you? Or the night before?) Or chicken noodle (using some of the pasta from when you had spaghetti recently). Begin to think of leftovers as a source and ally to your cooking and not a burden just to be reheated and eaten as is. Make a little extra, at times, of things you know you can use up handily and in a variety of ways. Don't make everything into an omelet or you'll never want to see another very soon. It's lucky soups are so ideal for using up leftovers, since all but soup haters can usually face it on quite a regular basis. All kinds of little odds and ends can be recycled here. Get in the habit of saving everything, no matter how small. Save it properly, however. Food poisoning is a concern here as anywhere. If you're not going to use something right away, make a small package and label, date, and freeze it. If things start to pile up, make soup.

2. Make everything from scratch so far as is possible. For example, pasta from a box and sauce from a jar is not exactly homemade, but it's several steps closer to homemade than a frozen spaghetti dinner that works out to ten times the price (and at very little savings of convenience). Convenience foods do have their place, but use them wisely. Many sauces are now available that you can just spoon over a chop or chicken breast and run into a hot oven. Or toss onto pasta. Again, though these things are far from truly homemade, they are *much* cheaper than the alternative of takeout food.

For the greatest savings, learn enough about cooking so that you can really make things from scratch. A hearty bean soup can be made for literally pennies a serving; "to go" or "heat and serve" that same soup might cost from .75 to $1.50 or more! You can also freeze some and save it for later as a convenience food.

For another easy, dramatic example: Price a takeout roast chicken and estimate its size. Then compare the cost of a similar-sized chicken in the meat counter of your market. Even if the chicken is not on sale, the cost difference is apt to be $6.00 versus $1.50. Nothing is simpler than roasting a chicken: put it in a pan, put it into a hot oven, come back in forty-five minutes to an hour. While you're at it, put two chickens in the pan and later have chicken salad, chicken pot pie, chicken and dumplings, you name it. The more nearly you begin from the beginning in cooking, the greater the savings are apt to be.

Beyond cooking from scratch and using up all leftovers, there are foods that are bargain bonuses well worth your attention.

EGGS

Eggs are an excellent and easily digestible protein source that lend themselves to a seemingly endless variety of preparations appropriate for morning, noon, and night. Books are devoted to this single mainstay ingredient. In addition to morning's scrambled and fried eggs, omelets make great entrees for lunch or supper. Eggs can be put into a small greased baking dish over some (leftover) vegetable or meat and baked for shirred eggs. These same ingredients can be whisked together with a little milk or half-and-half and baked in a crust for a quiche. Even a complicated-sounding soufflé is nothing more than egg whites separated from the yolks, whipped, and folded back together with a little flavoring and (you guessed it) any available leftover. The very finest cooking is frequently excellent ingredients simply prepared, and nowhere is this requirement more economically met than with fresh, cheap eggs.

BEANS AND LEGUMES

Along with rice, beans and legumes are the great economical protein food source. They are the mainstay of much indigenous cooking the world over and are delicious besides. Buying these in bulk is usually your best bargain. If you are not familiar with cooking beans and legumes, see page 165 for the simple underlying principles that make it easier and tastier.

PASTA

From lasagna, that great mainstay of student households, to spaghetti with meat sauce and a grating of cheese, pasta can be a great ally to the kitchen on a budget. Be mindful that the protein in wheat, while valuable, is incomplete and therefore requires complementing to be utilized by the body. With pastas this usually means adding a meat or cheese component such as is mentioned above. By itself spaghetti with a plain (vegetarian) sauce and no cheese provides virtually no usable protein.

TUNA

By the cost per grams of protein, canned tuna is one of the very best bargains going. If digesting fats is not a problem, tuna canned in oil is extremely calorie dense. If fats are a problem, tuna canned in water is still quite an economical source of high-quality protein. Tuna salad, tuna melts, tuna croquettes, and tuna casseroles are all obvious choices here. Also consider a fish soup using canned tuna or substituting tuna for clams for a pasta sauce.

Slowly but surely, adequate nutrition has come to be looked at as a right and not a privilege. In recognition of this fact, programs such as the food-stamp program have been instituted. If you qualify for these programs, use them! Such assists can make an enormous difference in the quality and amounts of food you are able to buy.

Adequate nutrition has also come to be viewed as an inextricable component of optimal health and to that end meals-delivery programs for people with HIV/AIDS have been developed in many places around the country. (A list of the major providers is included in Appendix B.) Beyond this, congregate meals programs are sponsored by many HIV (and other) service organizations, as well as food pantry programs, which distribute groceries. Make use of all of these programs, for that is why they exist.

Some people feel that by using such programs they are taking food out of the mouths of people who may need it more. As noble as that concern is, it is misplaced. In order to be a success, a program must be used. Successful programs tend to survive; programs for which there is not a clear and proven need tend to go under. The greater truth is that you may be *helping* ensure that others continue to get adequate nutrition who otherwise might not—simply by using the programs that are designed to help all of us. To see what may be available in your area, check with your nearest AIDS service organization.

Recipes

EASY SEASONINGS
  Many people draw an absolute blank when faced with a spice cabinet. For those people the difficulty of cooking is not the effort, but the knowing how to manipulate flavors to provide variety. A simple chicken breast can be different night after night with only the simplest of changes in seasonings. To this end there is a wealth of handy products that can streamline and enhance your endeavors.

  Spike
  Mrs. Dash
  Old Bay
    These are general, all-purpose seasonings, good with a wide range of foods, from soup to roast meats to sauces. They offer an easy balance of seasonings. Good to boost flavor.

  Worcestershire sauce
  soy sauce
    These add both depth of flavor and complexity to savory dishes.

Tabasco et al
> This and other red-pepper sauces add more than just heat, they add life to many foods, even when used so discreetly that you can't taste the heat.

Jane's Krazy Salt
lemon pepper
> For when you want more of a "punch" than the plain version will give you.

chili sauce
tomato paste
anchovy paste
> These sauces can be used to round out and strengthen flavors in many dishes: soups, salad dressing, marinades, sauces. Even for those who don't like anchovies, anchovy paste can be used in such discreet amounts that you would never recognize the anchovy taste, but will recognize a subtle richness of flavor for its addition.

vermouth, sherry, Madeira
> All of these will keep in the pantry indefinitely and can be used to give a pronounced wine flavor. In addition, vermouth is herb flavored and will lend an automatic seasoning to your dish. It has been said that if your sauce is missing a "certain something," nine times out of ten it is missing a tablespoon or two of Madeira. Please note that the trace amount of alcohol added by these seasonings evaporates almost instantly upon being heated.

orange marmalade
> Orange marmalade is not too sweet and can lend its zesty flavor to many dishes where you would not expect it, especially those with tomatoes. Try a tablespoonful heated into a serving of tomato soup or try it added to a marinara sauce.

flavored vinegars and oils

If vinegar adds tang to a dish, flavored vinegars add that much more. Balsamic and cider vinegars are good to have on hand, as well as red and white wine vinegar. If you want to explore further, sherry vinegar and rice vinegar have their own distinctive tastes. Beyond these, see recipes for "Flavored Vinegar" and "Flavored Oil" on pages 186 and 187.

HUMMUS

This favorite dip turns out to be yet another traditional complementary protein. Enjoy it with raw vegetables or toasted pita bread. A food processor or hand blender is definitely called for here.

*1 can (15 ounces) chick peas
  (garbanzo beans)
1/4 cup tahini (sesame seed
  paste found in specialty
  food counters and health-
  food stores)*

*1/4 cup olive oil
2 cloves garlic
1 tsp. salt
1 tsp. cumin
1 tsp. pepper
juice of 2 lemons*

Place garlic and salt in food processor; pulse. Add chick peas, tahini, cumin, pepper, and lemon juice. Pulse until thoroughly ground. Add olive oil and continue processing to a smooth paste.

SALMON SPREAD

Salmon and cream cheese are both great protein sources. This spread keeps well; have it on hand as a nutritious/high-calorie snack on crackers. A food processor, mixer, or a strong arm is called for here.

1 pound cream cheese	*1 Tbs. dill*
1 can (15 ounces) salmon	*juice of 1 lime or lemon*

BY MACHINE:
Allow cream cheese to come to room temperature. Drain salmon, discarding any skin or bones. Pulse/process or beat with mixer until finely shredded. Add dill and juice and mix. Add cream cheese and blend until a smooth paste results. Refrigerate.

BY HAND:
Allow cream cheese to come to room temperature. Drain salmon, discarding any skin or bones. Crush and work with the back of a mixing spoon until finely shredded. Add dill and juice and mix. Add cream cheese and beat until a smooth paste results. Refrigerate.

PIMENTO CHEESE

Pimento cheese is terrific on crackers, as a dip for raw vegetables, or as a sandwich. Also, don't miss it as a grilled cheese sandwich.

1 pound cheese (sharp
    Cheddar or Swiss)
3/4 cup mayonnaise

1 jar (4 ounces) diced
    pimientos
salt and pepper to taste

Grate cheese and stir in remaining ingredients. So easy!

᷍

EASIEST LIVER PÂTÉ

Make "Best Liver and Onions," page 181 (or make extra when you have it for dinner one night). Pulse/process everything in a food processor with a little extra salt and pepper until finely minced. Add 4 ounces cream cheese and process until a smooth paste results. Refrigerate. Have on crackers for an extra-nutritious snack.

OPTIONAL GARNISHES:
    Chopped onion
    Dill or sour pickle slices
    Whole-grain mustard
    Sliced hard-boiled egg

EGG DROP SOUP

per serving

Egg drops are an excellent nutritional add-on for broth (versus cream or hearty) soups. Traditionally they are made with chicken broth, but any will do. Egg drop soup is easier to make than scrambled eggs.

*1 cup broth (homemade or   1 egg
    canned)*

Bring broth to a full boil. Whisk egg with a fork, as for scrambled eggs. Stir broth with fork in a circular motion while pouring in egg. Remove from heat and serve immediately.

VARIATION:
Try this using a package of ramen noodle soup mix, such as Oodles of Noodles.

AVGOLEMONO

per serving

This classic Greek soup is like a refreshing breeze in summer and like a warming memory of summer in winter. This whole process takes only a few moments.

1 serving chicken-and-rice soup (homemade or canned)

juice of $\frac{1}{2}$ lemon
1 egg

Bring soup to a boil and add lemon juice. Whisk egg in small bowl until thoroughly beaten. Add a few ounces of hot broth while continuing to whisk. Add more hot broth until about $\frac{1}{2}$ of broth has been incorporated into egg. Return egg mixture to pan and stir constantly until thoroughly heated. Serve at once.

BEAN AND LEGUME COOKERY

Beans and legumes are a delicious and economical form of protein that many people avoid in the belief either that cooking them is mysterious or difficult or that flatulence is the irrevocable result of eating them. Neither of these things is true.

Many, many different types of beans and legumes are available, not to mention the almost endless combinations. A thirteen-bean soup is not rare! Experiment with different varieties to discover which you like best. Those bought in bulk or generic packages are your best bargain.

For all their variety the basic rules for cooking all beans and legumes are simple.

First, soak the beans or legumes overnight in water to cover (by several inches), then drain and rinse thoroughly in fresh water. This important preliminary will significantly reduce the starches that are the main culprits in causing gas. A slightly less acceptable (but much quicker) method is to bring the beans or legumes to boil in water to cover for one minute, allow them to sit for one hour, drain, and rinse in fresh water. Then proceed with the recipe.

Second, cook all beans or legumes over a gentle heat until they reach a desired state of tenderness BEFORE ADDING ANY ACID INGREDIENT such as vinegar or tomatoes. Acid will arrest the tenderizing process and no amount of cooking will help if you add the acid too early. Cooking usually takes an hour or two. Don't try to rush the process with a higher heat.

Beans and legumes can be bland, so don't be shy with flavorings. A good stock is a much better base for a soup than water. Instant bouillon is handy to punch up the flavor. Spices too; cumin is excellent and provides an earthy warmth sometimes missing from a cozy bean soup. A splash of dry sherry just before serving doesn't just add a delicious flavor and aroma; it also helps make many bean and legume soups more digestible.

If, even after the preliminaries of soaking and rinsing, you find that beans and legumes still don't completely agree with you, try eating them in smaller amounts but more often. As your digestive tract becomes more accustomed, you should find that you have less and less difficulty digesting them. Also, BeanO, a commercial enzyme product (which is made by the same company as and functions similarly to Lactaid) can help reduce digestive problems related to beans and legumes.

BEAN SOUP

serves 4–6

*1 pound beans/legumes
(singly or in any
combination)*
1 large onion
*3–4 cloves of garlic
(optional)*
1 Tbs. oil

*1 cup cooked ham, sausage, or
chicken*
                    or
2 ham hocks
2 bay leaves
stock or water
salt and pepper to taste

Soak beans overnight in water to cover. Drain and rinse thoroughly. In a large pot, sauté chopped onions and garlic in oil until very lightly browned. Add remaining ingredients except salt and pepper. Cover with stock or water. Bring to a boil, stir, and lower heat until barely simmering. Cook gently for 1–2 hours, until beans are desired degree of tenderness. Water may be added during cooking if soup becomes too thick. Add salt and pepper to taste. If ham hocks have been used, remove from soup during the last half hour of cooking; discard skin, fat, and bones and return meat to the soup.

VARIATIONS:
- Add chopped bell pepper or celery when sautéeing onion.
- Add thinly sliced carrot during last half hour of cooking.
- When beans have reached desired degree of tenderness, add a can of chopped tomatoes.
- Serve with a dollop of sour cream and a sprinkle of chopped onions.
- Serve with grated cheese.
- Add a spoonful of dry sherry to each portion just before serving.

GINGER SHERRY PORK CHOPS

per serving

This marinade is also great with boneless chicken breasts.

MARINADE:

1 Tbs. soy sauce
1/4 cup dry sherry
1 clove garlic

1 Tbs. honey
3–4 slices fresh ginger root

Combine the ingredients and warm to dissolve the honey. Place a thick-cut pork chop into the marinade for 20 minutes, turning once. Broil or grill.

⁓

ORANGE GLAZED CHICKEN

per serving

This chicken is easy and delicious. The sugar in the marmalade caramelizes as the chicken bakes, browning beautifully and dispelling any residual sweetness.

1 chicken breast
1–2 Tbs. orange marmalade

salt and pepper to taste

Preheat oven to 375°F. Place chicken breast skin side up in baking pan. Heat marmalade until syrupy and brush over chicken. Bake for 10 minutes and reglaze. Bake until chicken is done (about 35 minutes total for average sized breasts).

VARIATION:
• Substitute apricot preserves for marmalade.

SAVORY BREAD PUDDINGS

These are first cousins to quiches and even easier. They are a great way to use up old bread.

CHEESE CASSEROLE

4 servings

4 cups (about 6–8 slices) bread, diced

1 cup grated cheese (sharp Cheddar or a combination of Swiss or Gruyère and Parmesan)

2 eggs

1 cup milk

¼ cup noninstant powdered milk (optional—for extra protein)

salt and pepper to taste

several drops of Tabasco (optional)

3 Tbs. butter

Preheat oven to 350°F. Generously grease casserole dish with butter. Combine bread and cheese and place in baking dish. Beat to combine thoroughly the remaining ingredients and pour over bread and cheese in casserole. Dot top with any remaining butter. Bake about ½ hour until puffed and brown.

CHARLESTON SHRIMP PIE

4–6 servings

Another savory bread pudding, this time with no milk. Ham may be substituted for the shrimp.

4 cups (about 6–8 slices)
  bread, diced
1 pound cooked shrimp,
  peeled
1 small onion, chopped
1 small bell pepper, chopped
1 can chopped tomatoes

2 eggs
1 cup tomato or V-8 juice
1 Tbs. butter
Salt and pepper to taste
several drops of Tabasco
  (optional)

Preheat oven to 350°F. Toss together bread, shrimp, onion, bell pepper, and tomatoes and place in buttered casserole. Beat to thoroughly combine remaining ingredients and pour over bread mixture. Bake until puffed, crusty, and brown, about ½ hour.

BOILED CHICKEN

Boiling is an easy way to cook chicken, both as a preliminary step for other dishes and for its plain and simple goodness; ". . . as Queen Victoria used to have it!"

BASIC RECIPE:

1 chicken	*(optional) onion, celery, carrot,*
water	*bay leaf*
salt and pepper to taste	

Place the chicken (and optional onion, celery, carrot, and bay leaf) into a pot large enough to leave several inches of head room, barely cover with water, and place over a medium high heat. Allow to come to a boil and skim any scum that may gather at the top. Reduce heat to low and allow to simmer. Go about your business—sing a song or go to a movie. Stewing a chicken is a casual affair and may be made to accommodate your schedule completely. A slow cooker, such as a Crock-Pot, is ideal here. At some later time (anywhere from 1 to 8 hours later, depending on how tender you want the meat to be), remove chicken from the broth and allow it to cool until you can handle it. Remove the meat and return the skin and bones to the broth. Simmer for another couple of hours, then strain into a wide pot or deep pan and skim the fat from the surface. If you are being very careful to remove from your diet as much fat as possible, you may chill the broth, which will cause broth and fat to congeal in different layers; thus you can lift the fat from the top.

Enjoy your chicken as is or proceed with any of the following recipes. Use broth as chicken soup or as the base for other soups or white sauce.

CHICKEN SOUP

To the boiling broth from the boiled chicken (page 171), return some of the meat and either rice or noodles (these may be uncooked or leftovers) for chicken-and-rice soup or chicken noodle soup, respectively. Add salt and pepper to taste. Beyond that your imagination—and stock of leftovers—is the limit.

OLD FASHIONED CHICKEN AND DUMPLINGS

Though chicken and dumplings are made in many places using a noodlelike dumpling, these dumplings are like soft little clouds that enrich the broth and give it a soothing, creamy consistency (without cream). It is a favorite from my North Carolina childhood and the greatest comfort food I know, here revised slightly to increase its nutritional value.

BASIC RECIPE:

1 boiled chicken with broth   *salt and pepper to taste*
enriched formula biscuit
  dough (page 175)

Return the chicken meat to the broth, pulling the meat into shreds as you do. Cook this until the meat is as tender as you like (traditionally, the meat is cooked until it dissolves). This recipe may be made in advance to this point at any time convenient and refrigerated or frozen until needed.

To serve, bring broth (with meat) to a rolling boil and season to taste with salt and pepper. Drop biscuit dough by the heaping teaspoonfuls into the broth until the dumplings cover the surface in a single layer. As you do this, you will notice that the dumplings swell a great deal, so don't overcrowd. Cover the pot with a tight-fitting lid, reduce heat to low, and allow to cook for eight to ten minutes. Some of the flour will release from the dumplings, gently thickening the broth to form the lightest of gravies. Stir gently up from the bottom (where most of the meat will have settled) and ladle dumplings, meat, and broth into soup bowls. This dish may be gently reheated, but may need a bit of additional water stirred in, as it tends to thicken somewhat as it stands.

STREAMLINED VERSION:

cooked chicken
(approximately two cups
meat)—canned, leftover,
or deli takeout
1 large can (1 qt.) chicken
broth

1 cup instant baking mix (such
as Bisquick)
milk or water

Shred chicken meat into broth and boil until desired degree of tenderness. Using a casually measured cup of baking mix, add enough milk or water to make a sticky dough (exact proportions will vary slightly by brand). Continue with instructions on page 173.

BISCUITS

Due to the amount of fat in biscuits, they are really quite calorie laden, and since the fat is absorbed and emulsified by the flour, it is more easily digested than many fats encountered in less emulsified forms. In addition to the standard accompaniments of preserves or butter, biscuits are great with ham or sausage. Make a full-sized recipe and munch on cold biscuits through the day for lots of calorie add-on and good-quality protein from the enriched flour formula. By the way, though somewhat less nutritious, commercial baking mixes (such as Bisquick) make excellent biscuits and are very convenient if you're not feeling up to the "scratch" variety.

2 cups enriched flour (page 176)
1/2 tsp. salt
1 Tbs. baking powder
1/3 cup shortening, butter, or combination

1 cup milk (water may be substituted by the lactose intolerant)

Preheat oven to 450°F (it is important that the oven be hot when the dough goes in). Put dry ingredients into a large bowl and stir to thoroughly combine. Remove a good-sized handful to your work surface and add the shortening to the remainder. Work this into the flour with your hand, squeezing it through your fingers and mashing it against the bowl until it is thoroughly combined. Add the milk and stir in with a spoon (it will be very sticky) until just blended. Scoop out dough onto the reserved flour and go wash the bowl (giving the dough just a moment to rest). Turning the dough in the flour to coat its sticky surface, begin to knead the dough gently and briefly just until all of the flour is incorporated. Don't overdo it here or your biscuits will be heavy and dense. Drop biscuits are made simply by dropping heaping spoonfuls of dough onto a baking sheet (as with many cookie doughs).

Rolled biscuits, the more standard variety, are rolled with a rolling pin or patted out with the flat of your hand until the dough is approximately ½ inch thick and then cut into the shapes desired. (Should the dough still be too sticky to work easily, sprinkle extra flour to keep the surface of the dough manageable.) Though any drinking glass can be pressed into the surface to produce a round biscuit, the best biscuits by far are cut with a biscuit cutter or knife, as the cleanly cut edge allows the biscuit to rise to greater, lighter heights. Gently mass together scraps of dough, reroll, and continue until all dough is used. Bake until golden brown, approximately 10 to 12 minutes.

〜

ENRICHED FLOUR MIXTURE

The following formula is based upon the famous Cornell triple-rich flour formula and is an excellent nutritional enhancement to any of the purposes for which you may use flour. These additions do not change the cooking properties of the flour and it may be used in any recipe without adjustment. The presence of dairy should be noted by the *severely* lactose intolerant and be deleted (at nutritional sacrifice) if necessary.

5 lbs. unbleached, enriched flour
1¼ cups soy flour

1¼ cups dry powdered milk
⅓ cup wheat germ

Simply stir or sift together thoroughly these ingredients and keep on hand for all of your flour needs. Should your sieve be fine, many of the larger particles of wheat germ will not pass through and will need to be stirred back into the finished mixture. Soy flour may be found in many supermarkets and virtually all health-food stores.

QUICHE

serves 4

Quiches, with their endless variations, are a great way to use up leftovers. They are packed with nutrition and very easy to make if you begin with a premade crust.

Basic Quiche

9 inch pie crust
        or
8 inch deep-dish pie crust
2 cups milk
¹/₂ cup noninstant powdered
    milk (optional—for added
    protein)
3 eggs

²/₃ cup grated cheese (Swiss,
    mozzarella, Gruyère,
    Cheddar)
salt and pepper to taste
1 cup chopped or diced cooked
    meat or vegetable or any
    combination thereof

TRY:

- A combination of bacon and sautéed onions, using Swiss or Gruyère cheese
- Diced ham, using Swiss or Gruyère cheese
- Broccoli, using Cheddar cheese
- Chicken, using mozzarella

Preheat oven to 425°F. Prick pie crust all over with fork and cook until barely brown. If crust has bubbled up while prebaking, simply press gently back into place. While browning crust, beat together the milk, milk powder, eggs, and salt and pepper. Place cheese and meat and/or vegetables in crust, pour over custard mixture, return to oven, and immediately reduce heat to 325°F. Bake for 35 minutes or until a knife inserted into the center comes out clean. Serve warm.

FRITATA

2 servings

A *fritata* is an easy Italian omelet, which may be eaten hot, cold, or at room temperature. Eggs are about the best nutritional bargain going and this dish is an excellent way to use up leftovers.

6 eggs   salt and pepper to taste
1 Tbs. oil
1 cup cooked meat,
    vegetables, cheese, or
    combination

Preheat oven to 400°F. On top of stove, heat oil in an 8-inch heavy skillet until quite hot. Thoroughly beat eggs and add to pan—it will sizzle and form a skin around the bottom and sides. Distribute filling evenly over the bottom of pan and place in hot oven. Cook for about 10 minutes (exact time will vary depending on size and shape of pan, temperature of filling ingredients, et cetera). When no egg remains liquid, remove from oven and invert onto plate.

Hot: You might glaze the surface with a pat of butter.

Room temperature: Try this with a condiment such as salsa or have as a sandwich with lots of (flavored) mayonnaise.

Cold: Dice up omelet and add to a salad.

THE MEAT LOAF

A good meat loaf is perhaps the all-time great comfort food. It is also great food. With its uncanny ability to absorb random ingredients, you can pack in any number of nutritional add-ons or simply put many leftovers to good use.

A meat loaf is almost always an extemporaneous affair, with a dash of this and a touch of that. It would never occur to me to measure anything, and I give the following measures as indications of proportions only. The basic recipe below is just a starting point. Add to it whatever of the additions appeal to you, or anything else you can think of. Do not use the leanest meat for meat loaf or it will be dry and lacking in flavor. Choose ground round over ground sirloin.

Basic Meat Loaf

4 servings

2 pounds ground meat (beef or a combination of beef, veal, and pork)
1/2 cup seasoned bread crumbs
2 tsp. Spike (or other spice mix) or herbs to taste
salt and pepper to taste
1/2 cup Parmesan or Romano cheese, grated
1 egg
1 Tbs. Dijon mustard
1 Tbs. Worcestershire sauce
1 Tbs. soy sauce
1/2 cup ketchup

Preheat oven to 350°F. Mix together meat, Spike, salt and pepper, bread crumbs, and 1/4 cup cheese. Add egg, mustard, Worcestershire and soy sauces, and 1/4 cup ketchup. Continue mixing until thoroughly blended. Pack into baking pan that will contain the mixture at a depth of 2–3 inches. Smooth remainder of ketchup onto surface, dust with remainder of cheese, and bake until done. This will vary depending upon how thick in the pan your mixture is—usually 45 minutes to an hour is about right.

ADDITIONS:

- 1 clove finely minced garlic
- 1 small onion, chopped
- 2 hard-boiled eggs (chopped or whole—they will make a lovely pattern when the meat loaf is sliced if left whole)
- Substitute rolled oats for part or all of the bread crumbs
- $1/2$ cup noninstant powdered milk
- $1/4$–$1/2$ cup wheat germ
- Green peas, diced carrots, cooked mushrooms, chopped celery, corn, or any leftover vegetable you happen to have lying around
- Crumbled bacon

BEST LIVER AND ONIONS

per serving

Okay, Okay; I know a lot of you out there don't like liver (or don't *think* you do). However, liver is a mother lode of nutrition and is worth cultivating a taste for. And who knows? Perhaps you just haven't had it the right way yet. Calf's liver or chicken liver is the mildest.

2 strips bacon	Madeira (optional)
1 small onion	salt and pepper to taste
serving portion of liver	
(approx. 4 ounces, sliced	
½ inch thick)	

In a skillet, fry bacon until done. Remove and add sliced onion. Cook gently until very lightly browned. Push onions to sides of pan and add liver. Liver cooks quickly, so turn once and cook just until firm through (no "squishiness"). At the last moment, add a splash of Madeira. To serve, pile onions on top of liver and top with bacon strips.

VEGETABLE CASSEROLE

4 servings

As a chef it is a great delight to serve to people foods they have never liked in forms that they find they love. The recipe that follows is a standard in the South, though it seems comparatively unknown north of the Potomac. One MANNA kitchen volunteer took this recipe home and served it to her husband—a man who had never willingly eaten squash in his life—whereupon he exclaimed, "This is the best chicken you've ever made!"

Though summer squash is the traditional vegetable used, many others may be substituted. Try using all onions.

*4 medium summer squash
(yellow squash), sliced—
about 4 cups
1 medium onion, diced
1/2 cup flour
1 cup Parmesan cheese*

*(optional) 1/2 cup noninstant
powdered milk for extra
protein
2 cups sour cream
3 Tbs. butter
salt and pepper to taste*

Preheat oven to 350°F. Mix squash and onion together and add flour, 1/2 cup of Parmesan cheese, powdered milk, and salt and pepper. Stir thoroughly to heavily dredge the vegetables. Stir in sour cream and turn mixture into buttered baking dish, press into place, and sprinkle remaining Parmesan cheese on top. Dot with any remaining butter and bake for 30 minutes or until squash is tender.

HOPPIN JOHN

serves 4

Of Charleston origin, this standard of my southern childhood is another example of a complementary protein dish. If the peas and rice are cooked together, as is sometimes done, the result is an unappetizing gray. I prefer the method below.

1 cup cooked rice   *3 strips of bacon*
2 cups dried black-eyed peas

Soak, drain, and rinse black-eyed peas as described on page 165. Barely cover with fresh water, add bacon, and simmer, covered, until tender. There should be no "crunch" left, but peas should remain individual, not be cooked to mush. Drain peas and discard bacon, but reserve about ¼ cup of cooking liquid. Return to pan with cooked rice, stir together, add reserved liquid, and heat gently for 5–10 minutes.

SUCCOTASH

This traditional vegetable combination of corn and lima beans has been a standby for over two hundred years that we know of. Of native American origin, it is an excellent example of how every culture instinctively develops complementary protein combinations.

Succotash generally comes to us frozen, with instructions for boiling. Instead, try thawing it first and sautéeing it in butter just until thoroughly hot. Add a hearty sprinkling of lemon pepper and stir for a minute longer. Many people who think they don't like succotash find that they love it when prepared this way. The lemon pepper makes the difference.

WHITE SAUCE

per cup

White sauce is the mother to many other sauces and dishes. It can easily take on a variety of flavorings and add nutrition, calories, flavor interest, and moisture to a variety of dishes. A little white sauce stirred into leftover peas becomes creamed peas. When made with beef stock and flavored with a tablespoon of Worchestershire sauce, it can be a gravy for reheated meat loaf. With a little cheese stirred in, it becomes a Mornay sauce, wonderful over vegetables or a baked potato. With a little more cheese stirred in, it is the base for macaroni and cheese. You can easily see how handy this can be to have around. White sauce will keep up to a week covered in the refrigerator, so try making two or three times the basic recipe and flavoring portions of it with any of the easy seasonings listed on page 158.

Instant-dissolving flours, such as Wondra, are specifically milled to make sauce making extra easy. If you find that you use white sauce often, make up a batch of enriched flour using instant-dissolving flour measure-for-measure and reserve it just for sauce making. The technique for making white sauce using instant-dissolving flour is a little different—and easier—so follow the package directions.

2 Tbs. butter

2 Tbs. enriched flour (page 176)

1 cup liquid (milk, half-and-half or stock)

1/4 cup noninstant powdered milk (optional—for extra protein)

salt and pepper to taste

Melt butter in pan over medium heat and add flour. Stir with a whisk to form a paste and continue stirring for a minute or two, making sure that no lumps remain and that the paste (roux) does not brown. Add liquid a few ounces at a time and whisk in thoroughly until all is absorbed. Turn heat to lowest setting and continue to stir for another minute. Allow sauce to cook gently for about ten minutes, stirring frequently. Add salt and pepper to taste.

- Chipped beef heated in white sauce becomes creamed chipped beef—try it on toast.
- Stir in chopped hard-boiled eggs and have over toast.
- Add an ingredient such as corn and more liquid to make a cream soup such as cream of corn.

FLAVORED VINEGAR

Having an assortment of flavored vinegars on hand can simplify your salad-dressing- and marinade-making. They can enhance other foods too. Try making potato salad with chive and sage-flavored sherry vinegar (go easy on the sage). With ease, you can have at your fingertips a variety of flavors to play with—some of them which might be difficult to incorporate any other way. Also, it's *much* less expensive to make your own than to buy flavored vinegars.

1 quart vinegar
¼ cup firmly packed fresh herbs (singly or in combination)
or
2 Tbs. dried herbs

or
¼ cup thinly sliced fresh ginger root
or
5 cloves of garlic, crushed

Simply add the flavoring ingredients to the vinegar and wait. Give the bottle a shake once in a while in passing. For herb vinegars, steep about two weeks. For ginger or garlic vinegar, about two days. Don't let it go longer, or the organic material can begin to break down. After the steeping time is up, strain the vinegar and keep it in a tightly closed bottle indefinitely. Add back a fresh piece of your flavoring ingredient, if you like, as an identifier, or label.

Tip: Don't go crazy with the complexity of your combinations. Two to three flavors is about as far as you can go without reaching a muddle. Remember: You can always combine the finished vinegars.

Buy vinegar in a quart bottle and pour off some into a measuring cup (for pouring ease). Force your flavoring ingredient into the bottle and refill with reserved vinegar (there will be a little left over).

FLAVORED OIL

Much like flavored vinegars, oils can be infused with flavor-ings, though the flavoring ingredient usually needs to be of a more robust character.

> 2 cups oil
> flavoring ingredient(s), see
>   below

Place oil and flavoring into a saucepan and heat oil slowly until just too hot to touch. Turn off heat, cover pan, and allow to cool to room temperature. Strain oil into tightly capped bottle, adding back a few pieces of your flavoring ingredient as an identifier. No need to wait—flavored oils are ready to use as soon as they are cool.

> 5 cloves garlic
> 1/4 cup fresh rosemary
> 2 Tbs. black peppercorns
>
> 1 Tbs. red pepper flakes
> 2 Tbs. caraway seeds

FOUR SEASONAL CHUTNEYS

Fruit chutneys are a wonderful way to play with flavors and add life to familiar foods. Where would the Thanksgiving turkey be without cranberry relish? The following recipes were offered by my friend, Greg Funk, who has a great talent for these wonderful condiments. Try them with plain grilled meat, poultry, or fish.

Basic Recipe

1 Tbs. oil
2 cups onion, chopped
2 cups Granny Smith apples,
   peeled and chopped
1 cup white raisins

2 cups sugar
1/2 cup vinegar
1 tsp. salt
1/2 tsp. pepper
1/2 tsp. red pepper flakes

Heat oil in large, heavy saucepan. Add remaining ingredients and simmer on medium heat 15 minutes until apple and onion begin to soften. Add fruit and seasoning from the seasonal choices. Reduce heat and simmer until fruits are cooked and liquids have reduced and thickened. Stir often at this point (the last 10 minutes or so) to keep from scorching. Cool and store in refrigerator.

SPRING ADDITIONS:
   4 cups rhubarb, chopped
   1 cup red raspberries
   zest of 1 orange
   2 Tbs. fresh ginger, peeled and chopped

SUMMER ADDITIONS:
   4 cups blueberries
   2 Tbs. chili powder
   zest of 2 lemons

FALL ADDITIONS:
   4 cups cranberries
   zest of 1 orange
   1 Tbs. juniper berries, crushed

WINTER ADDITIONS:
   4 cups pineapple, peeled, cored, and chopped
   1 Tbs. curry powder
   zest of 2 limes
   2 Tbs. whole mustard seed

CUSTARDS

Custard, which is simply cooked milk and eggs, comes to us in many forms, from dessert to the ubiquitous quiche of the 1970s. In addition to being delicious in all of their guises, they are highest-quality protein at lowest cost.

Baked Custard

serves 4

2 cups milk
1/2 cup noninstant powdered milk (optional—for added protein)

1/3 cup sugar
1/2 tsp. vanilla
pinch salt
2 eggs

Preheat oven to 325°F. Stir together all ingredients until mixed thoroughly. Pour into four individual baking cups or one baking dish. Place in a larger baking dish with hot water up to the level of the custard. Bake just until a knife inserted in the center of the custard comes out clean (about 45 minutes for individual cups, an hour for single casserole). Remove from hot water bath to cool. Chill and serve cold.

VARIATION:
- For rice pudding, stir 1–2 cups cooked white rice and an (optional) 1/2 cup raisins into custard mixture before baking. Divide into six individual baking dishes. When cold, dust lightly with cinnamon.

CHEESECAKE

10 servings

Cheesecake may be the perfect food. It is loaded with high-quality protein, packed with nutrition, and dense with calories. It is also much easier to make than almost anyone would believe and is great to keep around for a best-quality snack. If you find you make it often, check around for cream cheese sold in bulk, which is much cheaper.

graham-cracker crust (recipe
   page 192)
1 pound cream cheese
$^1/_2$ cup sugar
3 eggs

$^1/_2$ tsp. vanilla
$^1/_2$ tsp. salt
sweetened sour cream (recipe
   page 192)

Preheat oven to 325°F. Line bottom and sides of a nine-inch springform pan with graham-cracker crust. Soften cream cheese and beat in sugar. Add remaining ingredients and mix thoroughly. Bake for 30 minutes. Turn off oven and allow to bake for 15 minutes more. When completely done, the cheesecake should have no sheen to its surface. Remove from oven and allow to cool completely to room temperature (this will take several hours). Don't worry about any cracks or crevices that may develop during cooling: they will never be seen again. Reheat oven to 425°F. Spoon on sweetened sour cream and spread not quite to the ridge which has formed as the cheesecake has cooled. Bake for 10 minutes, cool, then refrigerate for at least one day before slicing.

SWEETENED SOUR CREAM

So easy, but so, so good. Try this anywhere you might use whipped cream: on fruit, on cake, dip cookies into it, dip your fingers into it. (I have a hard time not just sticking my face into it!)

2 cups sour cream   *1/2 tsp. vanilla*
1/4 cup sugar

Stir together and apply where it will do the most good.

ᕗᙏᕲ

GRAHAM-CRACKER CRUST

9 inch springform pan

Graham flour is simply whole wheat flour, championed by a health-through-nutrition enthusiast of the nineteenth century, Dr. Sylvester Graham. Known to us most as graham crackers, they are whole-wheat crackers sweetened and flavored with cinnamon.

1 1/2 cups graham cracker   *1/2 cup powdered sugar*
* crumbs*   *2/3 cup butter*

Allow butter to come to room temperature. Stir together crumbs and sugar. Add butter and knead together until a solid mass forms (the heat of your hands will help melt the butter slightly.) Press evenly onto bottom and sides of springform cake pan and refrigerate until needed.

SPICY GINGERSNAPS

³/₄ cup butter
2 cups light brown sugar,
    packed
2 eggs
¹/₂ cup molasses
2 tsp. cider vinegar

3³/₄ cups enriched flour (see
    page 176)
1¹/₂ tsp. baking soda
2 Tbs. ginger
¹/₂ tsp. cinnamon
¹/₄ tsp. cloves

Preheat oven to 325°F. Cream together butter and sugar. Add eggs one at a time. Beat until incorporated, then add molasses and vinegar. Sift together remaining ingredients and mix until well blended. Form dough into 1-inch balls and bake on a greased baking sheet for 10–12 minutes.

EXTRA-HIGH-PROTEIN PEANUT BUTTER COOKIES

1 stick butter
³/₄ cup peanut butter
1 egg
1 cup sugar (light brown for
    extra flavor)

¹/₄ cup milk
3 cups enriched flour (recipe,
    page 176)

Preheat oven to 325°F. Cream butter and sugar together. Mix in peanut butter, then egg. Beat in half of the flour, all of the milk, and then the remaining flour. Roll into 1-inch balls and bake on cookie sheet for 10 to 15 minutes.

FRUIT GELATIN

For everyone who remembers gelatin desserts only as bad days in the grade-school cafeteria, it may come as a surprise that gelatin can be quite delicious when made with real fruit juice.

1½ cups fruit juice
¼ cup cool water

1 Tbs. or 1 envelope unflavored gelatin

Sprinkle gelatin onto the water and allow to sit for 10 minutes. When gelatin has softened, warm over a gentle heat until just melted. Stir into fruit juice and refrigerate until set.

VARIATION:
- When gelatin is still "slushy" but not yet set, whip with a mixer and add a cup of yogurt and ¼ cup noninstant milk powder.
- Using orange juice, fold in 2 cups whipped cream when gelatin is still "slushy" but not yet set for a wonderful orange Bavarian cream

BLENDER DRINKS

For ease and speed of preparation, blender drinks can't be beat. They offer a nutritious alternative to "junk food" snacks and can help you add lots of extra calories to your diet. Use either a traditional blender or a hand blender in its accompanying beaker.

Flavoring syrups, such as those made by Torani, come in an array of flavors, from anise to passion fruit to tamarind. Frequently seen in coffee bars, these syrups are also widely available in specialty food stores. They are a handy way to constantly vary the taste of your blender drinks.

Never use raw eggs in blender drinks, as salmonella poisoning could result.

CREAM OF BANANA SHAKE

1 cup milk
¼ cup noninstant milk
  powder
1 ripe banana
2 Tbs. honey or sugar
½ cup yogurt

Blend to a smooth consistency.

VARIATIONS:
- Substitute a large ripe peach for the banana.
- Substitute fresh or frozen strawberries or raspberries for banana.
- Substitute half-and-half for milk for extra calories.
- Substitute sour cream for yogurt.
- Add ¼ tsp. cinnamon.

PEANUT BUTTER CUP SHAKE

1 cup milk
1/4 cup noninstant milk
   powder
1/2 cup sour cream

1/4 cup sugar
2 Tbs. cocoa powder
1/4 cup peanut butter

Place milk, milk powder, and sour cream in blender jar. Stir together sugar and cocoa powder (this will prevent the cocoa powder from lumping), and add to blender; then peanut butter. Blend to a smooth consistency.

VARIATIONS:
- Substitute cottage cheese for sour cream.
- Substitute half-and-half for milk for extra calories.

LACTOSE-FREE FRUIT SHAKE

1 cup fruit juice (orange,
   grape, apple)
1/2 cup soft tofu

2 Tbs. honey or sugar
1 ripe banana
2 ice cubes

Blend thoroughly until contents are smooth and ice cubes are pulverized.

LACTOSE-FREE "MILK" SHAKE

1 cup enriched rice drink
   milk substitute
$^{1}/_{2}$ cup soft tofu
2 Tbs. sugar or honey
2 ice cubes

$^{1}/_{4}$ tsp. vanilla extract
           or
2 Tbs. flavoring syrup (see
note page 195)
           or
2 Tbs. cocoa powder

Blend thoroughly until contents are smooth and ice cubes are pulverized. If using cocoa powder, mix first with sugar to prevent lumping.

NUTRITIONAL SUPPLEMENT ENHANCEMENT

Let's be frank: The problem with liquid nutritional supplements is their taste. The following are some suggestions for how to make them much more palatable than straight-from-the-can, without adding difficult-to-digest fats or compromising their valuable lactose-free status.

First, drink them cold, cold, cold. That alone will help a lot.

Second, consider the following ways to enhance or mask their flavor:

Extracts: Simplest of all, try using flavoring extracts commonly used for baking. A few drops of peppermint extract, rum extract (which is nonalcoholic), and almond extract all work well with both the chocolate and vanilla flavors of supplement.

Cinnamon and Cocoa: Or try a little cinnamon or extra cocoa powder. To make these blend in without clumping, first stir the powders into a spoonful of sugar before adding to the supplement. Don't be shy with these additions: a hefty dose of extra cocoa powder will make a pleasant bittersweet chocolate drink.

Maple: Maple syrup can also be used to flavor these supplements.

Flavoring Syrups: Coffeehouses and coffee bars abound and virtually all of them have an array (usually over two dozen!) of concentrated flavoring syrups. A typical brand is Torani. The range of flavors is spectacular. Due to their increasing popularity, they are also more and more widely available through specialty food stores. (If you can't find them through a regular retail store, see if your local coffeehouse will sell you a bottle.)

Lemon Juice and Flavored Vinegars: The nutritionally potent medium-chain triglycerides in virtually all liquid nutritional supplements also have a potent flavor (think: cod liver oil). What do you do when you have a fishy tasting piece of fish? Add lots of lemon! Some acid sharpness is what these beverages sorely need. Though this needs to be done in a blender to prevent curdling, it is one of the best flavor enhancers. Raspberry or blueberry vinegar is what is called for here—not herbal vinegars, such as terragon.

> *1/4 cup flavored vinegar or juice of 1 lemon*
> *1/4 cup sugar*

Blend briefly and drink immediately.

(Raspberry vinegar can be purchased or it can easily be made by steeping 1 package of frozen raspberries in 1 pint of white vinegar. Strain after 2 days and discard raspberries. This is important for reasons of food safety.)

Nonfat Sorbets: Excellent nonfat, nondairy sorbets are now made by both Häagen-Dazs and Ben & Jerry's that have clear, intense flavors. Other brands tend to have *much* weaker flavor intensity and are proportionately less successful.

Most recipes for masking a supplement's flavor with sorbet suggest blending it in a blender. Let me suggest an alternate technique. Add a scoop of sorbet to a serving of supplement and instead of blending, stir it in until almost—but not quite—thoroughly melted. Then drink the supplement and (if you've done this right) your last gulp will be a soft little lump of sorbet—a final burst of pure flavor that will clean your palate and leave a pleasant taste of its own lingering in your mouth.

Häagen-Dazs:
  Mango
  Raspberry
  Orchard peach
  Zesty lemon
  Chocolate
  Strawberry

Ben & Jerry's:
  Purple passion fruit
  Strawberry kiwi
  Piña colada
  Lemonade
  (Mocha not suggested)

Frozen Juice Concentrates: These are even more potently flavorful than sorbets. Use them in their unreconstituted forms.

Tropicana Twisters
  Orange strawberry
  Banana orange raspberry
Margarita mixes
Strawberry daiquiri mix
Limeade
Fruit punch
Five Alive
Raspberry lemonade
Orange juice
Grape
Cranberry
Dole
  Orange pinapple
  Pineapple
(Apple or grapefruit not suggested)

IMPORTANT NOTE ON CHOICES OF FLAVORINGS

Perhaps the greatest hurdle in finding acceptable flavorings to mask the taste of these supplements is to find ones that don't disappoint. In taste tests the orange flavor is usually the least popular because we all know what an orange tastes like and this sure isn't it. Instead, as you add flavors, try ones you're less familiar with. Do you really know what passion fruit tastes like? Try the Ben & Jerry's purple passion fruit sorbet. Have you ever tried tamarind? It is a widely available flavoring syrup, though relatively few outside the Latino community are familiar with its taste. Consider the Häagen-Dazs mango sorbet over the orchard peach. Of course, all of these flavors, familiar or not, can help add variety. Look around to see what suits you best. Just don't give up if your favorite flavors don't fill the bill (for the very reason that they are your favorites and you know them so well).

On a slightly different tack, flavor combinations can be both delicious and unique, so that our familiarity with their precise taste is less exact. Consider the strawberry kiwi sorbet. Or Five Alive juice concentrate. Or come up with your own new combinations.

PART FIVE

Further Thoughts

Suggestions for Helpers

Perhaps the greatest single point to be made to a person who would offer assistance to someone with AIDS, whether a simple trip to the store or actual bedside nursing care, is that, first and foremost, the individual's dignity and sovereignty *must* be respected. Failing that, the assistance that *is* rendered may only serve to exacerbate a sense of helplessness and loss of control that comes with facing any life-threatening illness. So profound are these issues that it is not rare for individuals to reject treatment regimens and face consequences almost certainly catastrophic, merely in an effort to regain control of their lives and to actively determine their destinies. Efforts, however well intended, that spring from some notion that you know better than the person living with HIV must be resisted. Bring cheer, yes. Encourage, yes. Manipulate or control, no.

Next, respect your own dignity. Some well-meaning caregivers self-effacingly assume that all stress and pain are with the person suffering from AIDS. HIV, in fact, affects us all. While the adage "Serve first those who suffer most" is correct, the admonition only directs us where to begin our efforts. As in much of life, we can only be loving caregivers if we are able to love ourselves throughout the process. Failing that, we are merely slatterns at the whim of someone whose demands may become inappropriate as a result of a distorted perspective borne of being surrounded by constant subservient behavior.

Assuming, then, a considered regard for human dignity all around, where to begin? Though the subject of this book is nutrition, the matter of being a helpful caregiver is much wider than simply that. No single issue exists in a vacuum.

LISTEN!

Sometimes it is all you *can* do and sometimes it is enough. Many people feel that they are up against the clock and that they simply haven't had a chance to tell their story. Don't mistake that the story is linear and didactic. Our "story" is frequently simply that which we tell and that which someone hears. In listening, you may gain important clues as to what is important to the person for whom you are caring and how best to serve him. This may include foods that he likes and doesn't like and foods that may or may not have agreed with him (even when he himself has not noticed the link). He may remember certain foods fondly, or happy situations of which food was an important component. The answer to the question "What was the best thing you ever ate?" may be more instructive than "What would you like for lunch?" It may also be the springboard for meaningful communication. Being a good listener does not mean sitting in stunned silence. It is possible to express interest without prying. Never to refer to the disease is to fall into the elephant-in-the-living-room trap, where everyone is conscious of its looming presence but no one is mentioning it. Such reticence can serve to deny the person living with AIDS the opportunity to broach the subject for fear that it is unwelcome.

OBSERVE!

Is the kitchen sink full of dirty dishes and the countertops a mess? Surely few things more discourage even the simplest food preparation. Don't feel you must always ask what needs to be done, when the answer is obvious. Depression and apathy may cause a person not to care whether the kitchen is cleaned, who might brighten at the prospect of order and harmony.

INCLUDE THE PERSON IN YOUR LIFE

Ask if she'd like to go along while you go to the plant store, drop off the kids, pick up the laundry. Too often people feel as though they have been shut away from the business of living and are forgotten. Engage them! Such involvement in life can do wonders for depression and for appetite. Simply watching television together can supply needed companionship.

ENCOURAGE PARTICIPATION AND DECISION MAKING

This issue of control/lack of control cannot be overstated. Consult with the person you would help and rough out several days' menus. Then inventory the pantry and make a shopping list based on her eating habits (not yours). Share the effort and activity of making a batch of cookies rather than simply appearing at the door with them or making them in the kitchen while your charge is at the other end of the house, perhaps feeling isolated.

TOUCH!

Feelings of isolation can be most palpable when we feel alone in our skin. There is nothing pitiable in the need to be touched: it is one of our most human needs. A hug or a back rub can make us feel cared for beyond anything. Be generous and loving in your impulses to touch, but not gratuitous. Remember that all people do not wish physical closeness from all others at all times.

Last, do not be afraid of the situation or of your own inadequacies. In all likelihood you have never been in this situation before and will benefit from some guidance. For specific and practical suggestions, review chapters 5 through 9 on food and water safety and be mindful that your own hygiene can impact greatly on someone living with AIDS. Also review Chapter 14, "Strategies

for Weight Gain and Maintenance." If your involvement is extensive, consider taking a home-care course from your local Red
Cross, AIDS service organization, hospice ([800] 658-8898), or
Visiting Nurses Association ([800] 426-2547). Understand, if
someone is peevish and testy, that it comes with the territory of
illness and may have nothing to do with you. Don't be afraid to
ask questions openly or state things frankly. "I don't know what to
do." "How can I help?" "I'm so sorry you're going through this."
Common sense, a kind heart, and an ability and willingness to see
things from the other person's point of view are the qualities that
make a valuable helper. If you are guided by love, have faith that
the rest will follow.

When Food Is Not Love

Death is a reality for everyone, but for some of us it is of more imminent concern. We live in a culture that by and large views death in simplistic fashion as something bad to be delayed and avoided at all costs. Yet death is one of the great chapters in our lives and consciousness of our own mortality is one of the few things that separate us from other animals. It is realistic to acknowledge that death may come to us as a friend to spare us from an existence reduced to anguish. The hospice movement is largely responsible for the growing awareness of enlightened care and pain management for those who are dying. This enlightened attitude extends to allowing people a compassionate and humane death.

As controversial as the deliberate precipitation of death may be, there is a vast difference between precipitating death and simply allowing it to occur. Life is impossible without adequate nutrition and hydration. At the end of life, whether through age or sickness, the natural course of progression to death is a shutting down. For most people (indeed, most animals), this means reducing or ceasing their intake of food and drink. Far from being an agonizing way to die, reduced hydration and nutrition is actually a natural and instinctive means of minimizing pain and anxiety. Sensory perceptions shut down, drowsiness takes over, and death is peaceful. To coerce or insist that a terminally ill patient be hydrated or fed (often intravenously) beyond realistic hope of recovery or meaningful life is to do him or her a grave disservice. Even the National Conference of Catholic Bishops, a group staunchly opposed to any notion of assisted death or suicide, has stated, "It can be good medicine and good morality to forgo artificial feeding when it can only impose additional burdens on a patient who is imminently dying from a progressive terminal illness."

The issue of determining the end of one's own life is a deeply personal matter and one that is much more rationally thought through in advance of crisis. For this reason the implementation of a living will is an effective exercise in sorting through the often conflicting thoughts surrounding what circumstances we wish for ourselves at the end of our lives. It is also the only way that we can legally ensure that our rights and wishes are known and respected.

Most controversial is the decision to precipitate the end of our own lives. Though many people think, *When things get bad, I'll just take rat poison,* the fact is, it often doesn't work that way. What may begin as a crisis visit to an emergency room becomes a lingering hospital stay, and though the likely outcome is obvious, the rat poison is not available. A dying person with the resolve may lack the means and therefore must prevail upon friends, family, or medical personnel to do that which is questionable ethically and legally: assist in a suicide. If precipitating your own death is your decision, **the option to refuse food and drink is always available to you.** The process is natural, is not painful, and is as reversible as any such undertaking ever is. It is the instinctual response in the natural world. As each of us has sovereignty over his or her own life, this most personal of decisions must be respected in the one to whom the decision matters most: the dying person.

Appendices

Appendix A
AIDS-Specific Meals Programs

Recognizing the importance of adequate nutrition in the presence of HIV, a number of AIDS-specific meals-delivery programs have been established in cities around the country. Some of these programs provide nutritional counseling and other services. Further, in many localities meals are delivered to people with AIDS by umbrella meals programs, such as those run by churches. If you do not live in an area serviced by one of the AIDS-specific meals-delivery programs listed below, check with your local AIDS service organization to see what is available in your area or with the National Association of Meal Programs at (703) 548-5558.

Beyond delivered meals, many, many AIDS service organizations around the country sponsor congregate meals for people living with HIV. These gatherings provide not only nutrition but also fellowship, fulfilling another of the criteria of long-term survivors: networking with other people with AIDS.

CALIFORNIA:
Project Angel Food
7574 Sunset Boulevard
Los Angeles, CA 90046
(213) 845-1800

Mama's Kitchen
1875 Second Ave.
San Diego, CA 92101
(619) 233-6262

Project Open Hand
2720 Seventeenth St.
San Francisco, CA 94110
(415) 558-0600

COLORADO:
Project Angel Heart, Denver Center for Living
915 E. Ninth Ave.
Denver, CO 80218
(303) 830-0202

CONNECTICUT:
Caring Cuisine, AIDS Project New Haven
Box 636
New Haven, CT 06503
(203) 624-0947

FLORIDA:
Cure AIDS Now
111 SW Third St.
Miami, FL 33130
(305) 375-0400

GEORGIA:
Project Open Hand
1080R Euclid Ave., NE
Atlanta, GA 30307
(404) 525-4620

ILLINOIS:
Open Hand Chicago
Suite 100
909 W. Belmont Ave.
Chicago, IL 60657
(312) 665-1000

LOUISIANA:
Food for Friends
2533 Columbus St.
New Orleans, LA 70119
(504) 944-6028

MARYLAND:
Moveable Feast
3401 Old York Rd.
Baltimore, MD 21218
(410) 243-4604

MASSACHUSETTS:
Community Servings
125 Magazine St.
Boston, MA 02119
(617) 287-1605

MINNESOTA:
Open Arms of Minnesota
P.O. Box 14578
Minneapolis, MN 55414
(612) 331-3640

MISSOURI:
Food Outreach, Inc.
Suite 309
4579 Laclede Ave.
St. Louis, MO 63108
(314) 367-4461

NEW YORK:
God's Love We Deliver
166 Avenue of the Americas
New York, NY 10013
(212) 294-8100

PENNSYLVANIA:
Metropolitan AIDS Neighborhood Nutrition Alliance
Box 30181
Philadelphia, PA 19103
(215) 496-2662

WASHINGTON, DC:
Food and Friends
Box 70601
Washington, DC 20024
(202) 488-8278

WASHINGTON (state):
Chicken Soup Brigade
1002 E. Seneca
Seattle, WA 98122
(206) 328-0171

CANADA:
A Loving Spoonful
(The Vancouver Meals Society)
Suite 100
1300 Richards Street
Vancouver, BC V6B 3G6
(604) 682-6325

Appendix B
800 (and other) Handy Reference Numbers

AIDS Clinical Trials Information Service
(800) TRIALS A

AIDS Prescription Project
(800) 227-1195

HIV-AIDS Treatment Information Service
(800) HIV-0440

American Dietetic Association
National Center for Nutrition and Dietetics
(800) 366-1655

AmFAR Treatment Directory
(800) 39AmFAR

Choice in Dying
(800) 989-9455

Dept. of Agriculture
Meat and Poultry Division
(800) 535-4555 (Ext. 0)

Environmental Protection Agency
Safe Drinking Water Hotline
(800) 426-4791

Food and Drug Administration
Food Labeling and Seafood Hotline
(800) FDA-4010

Gay Men's Health Crisis
(212) 807-6655

Hospice Link
(800) 331-1620

Indian AIDS Hotline
(800) 283-AIDS

International Bottled Water Association
(800) WATER11

National AIDS Hotline
(800) 342-AIDS
Spanish (800) 344-SIDA

National Association of Meal Programs
(703) 548-5558

National HIV-AIDS Treatment Info Line
(800) HIV-0440

National Hospice Organization Helpline
(800) 658-8898

National Minority AIDS Council
(800) 559-4145

National Pediatric HIV Resource Center
(800) 362-0071

National Sanitation Foundation
(800) 673-8010

Nutritionists in AIDS Care
(212) 439-8073

Project Inform
(800) 822-7422

PWA Coalition Hotline
(800) 828-3280

Visiting Nurses Association of America
(800) 426-2547

Appendix C
ACT UP Standard of Care

The ACT UP Standard of Care is published by ACT UP Philadelphia and is recognized nationally as the authoritative MINIMUM standard of medical care. Though this version is the most current as this book goes to press, the ACT UP Standard of Care is constantly revised and updated. For the most current version, write to:

ACT UP/Philadelphia
PO Box 15919
Middle City Station
Philadelphia, PA 19103-0919
(215) 731-1844
(215) 731-1845 FAX

The ACT UP Standard of Care is also posted on the Internet at:
http://www.critpath.org

HIV ADULT STANDARD OF CARE
POST-VANCOUVER EDITION
Version #9 July 23, 1996 by ACT UP/Philadelphia

For the ninth time, this Standard of Care—first conceived four years ago by Jonathan Lax (1949–1996)—is being revised and published to help insure individuals are getting a minimum level of care to maximize quality and length of life with HIV disease. This is a minimum standard. Many patients are asking for and getting a higher level of care from "the system." This standard is an adult standard: Children need a different standard due to different immunology threshold.

Big Name Panels Scramble to Set Standard for Use of New Protease Combo Regimens. . . . Although cautious optimism was the rallying cry for the eleventh International AIDS Conference in Vancouver, we were already well-grounded in the lore of good news from the protease inhibitor combination studies. Compounded with this was the word-of-mouth news from 100,000 individuals who are using the 3 approved protease drugs: saquinavir (Roche's Inverase™), ritonavir (Abbott's Norvir™), and indinavir (Merck's Crixivan™). We affirmed in our 8th Edition: "The prospect of leading edge care in the next year is tantalizing: a protease drug plus AZT/3TC combination, plus viral load measurements will be Standard of Care a year from now." Now a number of "official" panels are following our lead.

There was nothing in the Vancouver data to challenge our recommendations of nearly a year ago, but there was some refinement of the use of these drugs. **Saquinavir,** the least potent of the three drugs, has lower bioavailability—we await a new formulation. Coadministration with ritonavir increases blood levels, but even as it is being used in a number of practices, we need more data on toxicity and dosage (one early but somewhat disappointing report on this PI-PI combo was reported on at Vancouver). Grapefruit concentrate and ketoconazole also raise levels. In light of cross-resistance, a reasonable option: Start on saquinavir, switch to another protease when resistance develops. The dose is three capsules (600 mg) three times daily, with meals. **Ritonavir** is highly potent in raising CD4 counts, dropping viral load, and decreasing morbidity and mortality. It comes in 100 mg capsules which should be kept refrigerated, although single capsules can be kept for up to 12 hours at room temperature. It is poorly tolerated, with half of all users describing gastrointestinal toxicity and dropping the drug especially during the first two weeks. Interactions with many drugs commonly used by PWAs are a further problem—examine list of all coadministered drugs. Dose escalation from 5 to 14 days is recommended. It is highly cross-resistant with indinavir. **Indinavir** is highly potent (especially in retroviral naive persons—or in practice start a new retroviral combination, like AZT/3TC or d4T/3TC, when adding the protease) dropping viral loads to the undetectable range for 48 weeks and possibly much longer in virtually all persons studied. Indinavir should be administered as two 400 mg capsules every 8 hours, at least 2 hours after eating or 1 hour before eating. Persons should drink at least 2 to 4 liters of fluids per day to avoid kidney stones. The indinavir-AZT-3TC combination has relatively low toxicity, high potency, and lower cost than other combos, but may be highly cross-resistant with ritonavir. This combination may be considered in high risk occupational exposures to HIV. **Nelfinavir** (Agouron's Viracept) will be approved early next year.

Of course, 95% of the 10 to 100 million infected individuals in the year 2000 will not have access to these promising new drugs. We can get a man to the moon and back to earth safely, but can we get life-saving and life-enhancing drugs to those who need them?

Johns Hopkins' rules of thumb on use of protease inhibitors: 1. Never use monotherapy. 2. Don't add a protease inhibitor to a failing regimen. 3. Use full dose therapy. 4. Emphasize compliance. 5. Think about drug interactions. 6. Monitor viral load..

Viral load monitoring, although yet to be fully validated through clinical trials, is useful in guiding efficacy of combination therapies, when used in conjunction of CD4 tests which measure immune system competence: 1) We know little about absolute viral load, so look for changes in viral load of 1-log of greater; 2) Monitor frequently (every 3 to 6 months) to know if new treatments are effective; 3) Fight for insurance and Medicaid payments for these treatments; 4) Use with CD4 counts, but realize that short-term (8-week) increases do not necessarily signal better disease and survival prognosis. The pipeline now has new drugs (Nevirapine, the first non-nucleoside reverse transcriptase inhibitor, was recently approved) but many combos have yet to be tested. As we await integrase inhibitors, immune restorative and gene therapy strategies, several years down the road, we think out long-term treatment strategies carefully.

Don't Drink the Tap Water: The Philadelphia Water and Health Departments deny Philadelphia has a cryptosporidium problem despite proven water-borne outbreaks among PWAs (August 1994). They say "don't boil the water—you could burn yourself." Best: water filtered to an NSF 53 standard cyst removal. Or bottled water: Deer Park, Great Bear, Poland Spring, Naya, Saratoga, and Wissahickon are safe.

Good numbers to know: Philadelphia FIGHT: trials and treatment directory: (215) 985-4448. (Also look for FIGHT's excellent **Information You Need to Live** lecture series.) **NIH Trials** Information: (800) TRIALS-A. **We the People with AIDS:** (215) 545-6868 for a variety of services. **Critical Path AIDS Project:** 24-Hour Treatment Hotline: (215) 545-2212. Critical Path AIDS Project Internet web page: http://www.critpath.org (updated daily).

AND NOW A WORD FROM OUR SPONSOR: This standard, as always, is published as a labor of love by ACT UP/Philadelphia. No fancy government grants, drug company budgets, or opera/gala fund raisers. If you find this useful (or lifesaving) send us a sorely needed donation: ACT UP/Philadelphia, Box 15919, Philadelphia, PA 19103-0919. Phone: (215) 731-1844. Fax: (215) 731-1845. E-mail: pdavis@critpath.org. ACT UP meets weekly on Mondays at 7:30 P.M. at St. Luke and the Epiphany, 13th Street between Spruce and Pine, in Philadelphia. Copyright © 1996, Standard of Care Working Group. Authors: Jonathan Lax and Kiyoshi Kuromiya. Also available in Spanish. Reproduce for handouts.

WHEN PATIENTS TEST HIV POSITIVE AT ANY LEVEL OF T4 CELLS:

Baseline tests T4, %, and T8 ratio	Should be processed same day as blood is taken.
Baseline tests should also include:	Chemscreen, liver function, neuro test, urinalysis, CXR, and a baseline viral load (either Roche or Chiron, but stick with one or the other—the most sensitive one available).
Baseline Toxoplasmosis titer	If positive, follow carefully, monitor for symptoms.
Baseline ophthalmic eye tests	Build relationship with eye doctor. Learn to use Amsler grid at home.
Baseline dental exam	Fix gum and tooth problems. Regular dental care.
Baseline psychiatric exam	Some new "seropositives" need treatment for depression.
Anergy skin testing	Pneumovax inoculation if not previously inoculated.
Syphilis Test (use MHATP)	Overtreat with Benzathine Penicillin.
All patients	Consider flu shot each October, and H. Influenza shot.
Hepatitis A or B negative?	Consider Hepatitis A + B vaccination. 3-shot series.
Tuberculosis PPD test	If positive @ 5 mm, treat one year with INH + pyridoxine or Rifampin.
Herpes Zoster outbreak	Treat aggressively with acyclovir (Zovirax). Zoster is early symptom of HIV, occurring 3 to 5 years before other OIs.
Gynecological (vaginal, pelvic, breast) exams:	Every six months. Treat for candidiasis if present, topical cream, Diflucan, if it does not respond, consider diet changes (less dairy and sugar) and daily acidophilus.
Pap smear	Every six months. If abnormal (including atypia) follow with colposcopy and treatment. Treat any STDs.
Smoking, drugs, alcohol	Unhealthy, but no connection to long-term survival.

T4 ABSOLUTE COUNT* >500

T4/T8	Every 4 to 6 months; take test same time of day, send to same lab, process the same day.
Viral load test	Get baseline and monitor at appropriate intervals (3 to 6 months).
Office visit	Visual exam to include inspection of mouth and skin every 4 to 6 months.
Recurrent herpes outbreaks	Prophylax with acyclovir on a daily basis.
Pap smear	Every six months. If abnormal (including atypia) follow with colposcopy and treatment. Treat any STDs.
Dental exam	Exam and cleaning every 4 to 6 months to avoid infection.

Psychiatric	Continue counseling or join a support group. Exercise.
Research and reading	Become knowledgeable for upcoming decisions about antiviral therapy options.

T4 ABSOLUTE COUNT* 500–200

HIV Infection	Start antiretroviral therapy with ddI + AZT or AZT + ddC or AZT + 3TC if CD4 or % falls dramatically. Discuss treatment options with doctor—build partnership! If viral load progressively rises and CD4 drops by more than 20%, consider AZT + 3TC + Crixivan, or the relatively poorly absorbed Saquinavir. Or if access is a problem, consider protease inhibitor combination drug trial. If using an unresearched combo, monitor bloodwork closely for toxicities.
T4/T8 tests	Every three months, constant time and same lab.
Viral load	Test now become important in following disease and measuring antiviral efficacy (every 3 to 6 months). A 0.5 log drop in viral load means current regimen is working.
Anergy panel	Test functional immunity. Usually have to push for this.
PCP	If <300 T4 cells, and symptomatic, test for active infection by bronchoscopy. If asymptomatic do not begin prophylaxis until T4 cells <200 or % is below 1%.*
Pap smear	Test every 6 months. If abnormal (including atypia) follow with colposcopy and treatment. Treat STDs. Thrush (oral and esophageal). Local clotrimazole therapy (Mycelex); fluconazole (Diflucan) if treatment fails.
Dental	3 to 4 visits/year; treat long-standing problems. Possible ulcers or dry mouth. Treat gum problems.
Skin problems, foot fungus	See dermatologist; treat topically, aggressively.
Testosterone/hormone levels	Supplement with testosterone patches or shots if weight loss or (men only) loss of sex drive (test may not be necessary).
Expect sinusitis problems	Treat aggressively with decongestants and antihistamines. Watch for drug interactions. Have any pneumonia symptoms checked.
Nutrition inventory + Chemscreen	Treat nutritional deficiencies. Counseling and vitamins.
Exercise	Workout and train for strength, stamina, and building of lean body mass.

Psychiatric   Continue therapy or support group. Regular
                                     exercise.

T4 ABSOLUTE COUNT* 200–100

HIV infection   Continue therapy if chosen; switch to other
                                     combinations (AZT/ddC or AZT/ddI)if progressive
                                     viral load rise or T cell drop, and add indinavir.
                                     Frequent amylase levels if on ddI, watch for anemia
                                     if on AZT. AZT (and possibly Nevirapine) cross the
                                     blood-brain barrier—others don't. Use D4T or AZT
                                     plus 3TC plus saquinavir or indinavir as aggressive
                                     therapy with goal of reducing virus to undetectable
                                     levels. Acyclovir may have a survival benefit at 800
                                     mg/day. Monitor closely if using untested combo.
                                     Acyclovir has been shown in Australian studies to
                                     have survival benefit, use 800 mg/day. Monitor
                                     closely if using untested combo.

Viral load test   Very important for deciding when to switch therapies.

Candidiasis   Treat locally with topicals, fluconazole (safer), or
                                     ketoconazole.

PCP prophylaxis   Bactrim (Double Strength 3X per week) or aerosol
                                     pentamidine (with posturing) if unable to take
                                     Bactrim or dapsone. Add dapsone to pentamidine
                                     2X/week as adjunct if previous PCP patient.
                                     Bactrim is the preferred therapy (consider
                                     desensitization if Bactrim "intolerant"). Use
                                     Atovaquone (Mepron) as a backup.

Pap smear   Every six months. If abnormal (including atypia)
                                     follow with colposcopy and treatment. Treat any
                                     STDs. Candidiasis (oral, esophageal): Local
                                     clotrimazole therapy (Mycelex), fluconazole
                                     (Diflucan) if treatment fails.

Gynecological (vaginal, pelvic,   Every 3 to 6 months. Treat for candidiasis if
breast) exams: present, topical cream, Diflucan, if refractory,
                                     consider diet changes (less dairy and sugar) and
                                     daily acidophilus.

CMV   Continue eye exams; start gancyclovir or Foscavir if
                                     proven CMV infection. Treat aggressively. Jury still
                                     out on prophylaxis either oral gancyclovir and
                                     valacyclovir at this T4 count.

Toxoplasmosis   Titer once per year, if positive consider
                                     pyrimethamine prophylaxis; or with Bactrim.

TB   Any suspicions of TB should be x-rayed and
                                     cultured; treat very aggressively with 4 or 5 multi-
                                     drug therapy.

Office visit	Minimum every three months. Treat symptoms aggressively.
Hormone levels	Supplement testosterone (men only) if low. Deca-durabolin could be considered by women.
Fevers	Identify cause and treat. (Most people use too little Tylenol.)
Diarrhea	Treat with Imodium, but if it continues > 2 days, specialist must use full workup (not just stool exam, which won't always detect treatable MAI, CMV, Cryptosporidium, Microsporidium, Cyclospora, etc.) to diagnose cause. Treat aggressively.
Peripheral neuropathy	Best treatment is acupuncture (really), but some success with Tegretol or Elavil. Try oral niacin and B-12 shots.
Dental exam	Exam and cleaning every 4 to 6 months. Fix problems.
Nutrition and vitamins	Correct deficiencies, add vitamin and/or food supplements (Advera or Ensure) if there is weight loss.
Psychiatric	Continue therapy and/or support groups. Exercise important.

T4 ABSOLUTE COUNT* <100

HIV Infection	Continue antiretroviral therapy. Consider 3TC + AZT plus indinavir or ritonavir, or a drug trial. High dose (800 TID) acyclovir may have survival benefit at these levels.
Fungal prophylaxis	Fluconazole (Diflucan) 200 mg three times a week, but consider possible development of resistance.
Cryptococcal meningitis	Treat aggressively with Amphotericin B (liposomal formulations may be less toxic—less "shake and bake") + 5FC; prophylaxis with fluconazole to prevent crypto (but consider development of resistant fungi).
Toxoplasmosis	If positive, prophylax with pyrimethamine, Bactrim, or combo.
Candidiasis	Treat aggressively with fluconazole (Diflucan).
MAI/MAC	Consider prophylaxis with Biaxin (clarithromycin) (500 mg PO bid at lower dosage) or azithromycin (1200 mg PO weekly) if counts are < 75 CD4. Rifabutin (300 mg PO daily) as second line.
PCP (recurrent—moderate or severe)	After conventional treatment failure, use trimetrexate with leucovorin rescue as effective salvage protocol.

Cryptosporidiosis	Aggressive testing and treatment. Humatin works in some cases. But NTZ available at some buyers' clubs seems to be much more effective. Food/water, diaper-changing, and sex safety precautions.
Pap smear (women)	Every six months. If abnormal (including atypia) follow with colposcopy and treatment. Treat any STDs.
Wasting (10% body weight loss)	Serum albumin <3.0 is prognostic for wasting. Men should be on testosterone + nandralone therapy. Use medicinal marijuana (or Marinol—less effective) as appetite stimulant or for control of nausea. Check for undiagnosed infections, look for experienced specialist. Oxandlorone or deca-durabolin may be good options for women. Office visits monthly to bimonthly. Treat all other problems aggressively.

* T4 count is CD4 cell count. Practitioners should also count % of lymphocytes and treat accordingly. The 15% level is frequently considered a "trigger" for aggressive therapy even if CD4 >200. Many physicians consider % as important as absolute CD4 count. Delayed Hypersensitivity Skin Tests (DTH Anergy panels)—underadministered in the U.S.—are useful as functional test of immune system competence.

The following, while not part of the actual Standard of Care, can be useful to persons with HIV disease wishing to take some control of their health.

Finding, and keeping, a competent MD with AIDS treatment experience (and a "Just Do It" attitude) may be the single biggest factor in survival, according to recent studies. Stick with a medical practice with backup, so you can get care on evenings or weekends. Get second opinions. Review all medications taken so your doctor can help minimize side effects. Plan ahead.

SELF-MONITORING FOR OPPORTUNISTIC INFECTIONS:

Indication	Symptom	Action
CMV Retinitis	Sudden changes in vision; significant increase in floaters, distortion or absence of visual areas or fields	Get to an HIV-experienced opthalmologist—fast. Use Amsler grid at home for testing.
Cryptococcal Meningitis	Fever, severe headache, nausea, confusion, appetite loss, memory loss	Consult physician immediately.
MAI/MAC or TB	Fever, chills, malaise, weakness, weight loss, drenching night sweats.	Consult physicians. (Note: Diagnosis is frustrating and takes from 3 to 5 weeks.)

	(Cough in TB; abdominal cramps in MAC.)	
Toxoplasmosis	Dull constant headache, confusion, paralysis, fever, and neuro difficulties	Consult physician immediately.
Lymphoma	Mild fevers, quick swelling or enlarged lymph nodes, especially localized.	Physician should refer to HIV oncologist.
Kaposi's Sarcoma	Flat red to purple lesions anywhere on body, do not blanch when pressed	Physician should refer to dermatologist to biopsy.
PCP	Trouble walking up stairs, with breathing problems, moderate fever, fatigue, night sweats, dry cough.	Consult physician immediately.
Diarrhea	Often difficult to diagnose precise causes in chronic diarrhea.	Treat with Imodium. Consult physician for complete workup if lasts more than 2 days.
Anemia or Neutropenia	Absolute exhaustion, pale washed-out look.	Use EPO or Neupogen to restore.
PML	Severe mental problems—loss of cognition in late stage— fast progression, outlook poor.	Consult doctor. Reduce viral load aggressively with protease inhibitors, hope for remission.
Sinusitis	Common with HIV.	Treat with decongestants/ antibiotic.
Skin Problems	Common with HIV or with many drugs.	Consult dermatologist.
Foreign Travel	Watch food carefully. No unbottled water.	Consider Cipro prophylaxis.

NOTE: Some symptoms may be drug cross-reactions. State all drugs (dosage) being used to your doctor.

VITAMINS AND NUTRITIONAL SUPPLEMENTS:

People with HIV/AIDS often have reduced absorption of some micronutrients. People with HIV may want to consider taking a multi-vitamin (standard adult dose—Centrum Silver is good) plus the following supplements. Note: absorption of vitamins with food is uncertain.

Type	Dose	Reason
Vitamin C	2 to 5 grams per day as ascorbate.	Antiviral and anticancer proper-ties (unproven but this is widely used).
Beta carotene	25,000 to 30,000 IU daily.	Antioxidant. Raises CD4 count (?) Government studies dispute

		claims for heart disease and cancer.
Selenium	110 mg supplement daily.	Use in immune system; helpfulness unknown.
B Vitamins	Extra B vitamin tab daily.	May help with neuro problems or anemias.
B-12 Vitamin	Sublingual, IM injection, or intranasally.	May help with neuro—doesn't work when swallowed. May help with fatigue and liver problems.
Niacin	100 to 250 mg/day.	Can be helpful (with B-12 shots) for peripheral neuropathy.
Aerobic exercise	3 × 20 minutes/week.	Improves immune function.

ACT UP/Philadelphia has developed this information from sources believed to be accurate and reliable. However, ACT UP/Philadelphia and the members on its Science and Medicine Committee take no responsibility for treatment outcomes based on the information contained in this document. ACT UP does not treat patients. Patients must see a trained and competent MD for ongoing partnership in medical care.

Comments, updates, criticisms, and cash should be sent to ACT UP/Philadelphia, Box 15919, Phila., PA, 19103-0919. Phone: (215) 731-1844 or (215) 545-2212. E-mail: kiyoshi@critpath.org. Posted on Internet: http://www.critpath.org.

Appendix D
Living Will

Each state has different criteria determining what constitutes a legal living will. The following form is valid for New York state ONLY and is given as an example. For a living will to be valid, it <u>must</u> be specific to the state of your residence. Living wills for every state may be obtained through Choice in Dying (800) 989-9455.

INSTRUCTIONS
PRINT YOUR
NAME

PRINT NAME,
HOME ADDRESS,
AND TELEPHONE
NUMBER OF
YOUR PROXY

ADD PERSONAL
INSTRUCTIONS
(IF ANY)

© 1993
CHOICE IN
DYING, INC.

NEW YORK HEALTH CARE PROXY

(1) I, _____ hereby appoint:

(name),

_____
(name, home address and telephone number of proxy)
as my health care agent to make any and all health
care decisions for me, except to the extent that I
state otherwise.

This Health Care Proxy shall take effect in the
event I become unable to make my own health care
decisions.

(2) Optional instructions: I direct my proxy to
make health care decisions in accord with my
wishes and limitations as stated below, or as he or
she otherwise knows.

*(Unless your agent knows your wishes about artificial nutrition and hydration [feeding tubes], your
agent will not be allowed to make decisions about
artificial nutrition and hydration.)*

PRINT NAME, HOME ADDRESS, AND TELEPHONE NUMBER OF YOUR ALTERNATE PROXY	(3) Name of substitute or fill-in proxy if the person I appoint above is unable, unwilling, or unavailable to act as my health care agent.

_____

_____

(name, home address and telephone number of alternate proxy)

ENTER A DURATION OR A CONDITION (IF ANY)	(4) Unless I revoke it, this proxy shall remain in effect indefinitely, or until the date or condition I have stated below. This proxy shall expire (specific date or conditions, if desired): _____

_____

SIGN AND DATE THE DOCUMENT AND PRINT YOUR ADDRESS	(5) Signature _____

Date _____

Address _____

WITNESSING PROCEDURE

Statement by Witnesses (must be 18 or older)

I declare that the person who signed this document is personally known to me and appears to be of sound mind and acting of his or her own free will. He or she signed (or asked another to sign for him or her) this document in my presence. I am not the person appointed as proxy by this document.

YOUR WITNESSES MUST SIGN AND PRINT THEIR ADDRESSES © 1993 CHOICE IN DYING, INC.	Witness 1 _____

Address _____

Witness 2 _____

Address_____

Courtesy of Choice In Dying 11/93
200 Varick Street, New York, NY 10014 1-800-989-WILL

INSTRUCTIONS

NEW YORK LIVING WILL

This Living Will has been prepared to conform to the law in the State of New York, as set forth in the case In re Westchester County Medical Center, 72 N.Y.2d 517 (1988). In that case the Court established the need for "clear and convincing" evidence of a patient's wishes and stated that the "ideal situation is one in which the patient's wishes were expressed in some form of writing, perhaps a 'living will.' "

PRINT YOUR
NAME

I, _____, being of sound mind, make this statement as a directive to be followed if I become permanently unable to participate in decisions regarding my medical care. These instructions reflect my firm and settled commitment to decline medical treatment under the circumstances indicated below:

I direct my attending physician to withhold or withdraw treatment that merely prolongs my dying, if I should be in an **incurable or irreversible mental or physical condition with no reasonable expectation of recovery.**

These instructions apply if I am (a) **in a terminal condition;** (b) **permanently unconscious;** or (c) **if I am minimally conscious but have irreversible brain damage and will never regain the ability to make decisions and express my wishes.**

I direct that my treatment be limited to measures to keep me comfortable and to relieve pain, including any pain that might occur by withholding or withdrawing treatment.

While I understand that I am not legally required to be specific about future treatments **if I am in the condition(s) described above I feel especially strongly about the following forms of treatment:**

CROSS OUT ANY
STATEMENTS
WITH WHICH
YOU DO NOT
AGREE

I do not want cardiac resuscitation.
I do not want mechanical respiration.
I do not want artificial nutrition and
hydration.
I do not want antibiotics.

However, I **do want** maximum pain relief, even
if it may hasten my death.

ADD PERSONAL
INSTRUCTIONS
(IF ANY)

Other directions:

These directions express my legal right to refuse
treatment, under the law of New York. I intend my
instructions to be carried out, unless I have re-
scinded them in a new writing or by clearly indicating that I have changed my mind.

SIGN AND DATE
THE DOCUMENT
AND PRINT
YOUR ADDRESS
WITNESSING
PROCEDURE

Signed _____
Date _____
Address _____

I declare that the person who signed this document
is personally known to me and appears to be of
sound mind and acting of his or her own free will.
He or she signed (or asked another to sign for him
or her) this document in my presence.

YOUR WITNESSES
MUST SIGN AND
PRINT THEIR
ADDRESSES
© 1993 CHOICE
IN DYING, INC.

Witness 1 _____
Address _____
Witness 2 _____
Address_____

Appendix E
Additional Information

INTERNET:
A world of constantly updated information is available via the Internet: http://www.critpath.org

HIV/AIDS PUBLICATIONS:
The AIDS Treatment News
P.O. Box 411256
San Francisco, CA 94141
(415) 255-0588

BETA (Bulletin of Experimental Treatments for AIDS)
1250 Forty-fifth St., Suite 200
Emeryville, CA 94608-2924
(800) 959-1059

Critical Path AIDS Project Newsletter
2062 Lombard St.
Philadelphia, PA 19146
(215) 545-2212

POZ Magazine
P.O. Box 1965
Danbury, CT 06813
(800) 883-2163

GENERAL:

Brody, Jane E. *Jane Brody's Nutrition Book.* New York: W. W. Norton & Co., 1981.

Davis, Adelle. *Let's Cook It Right.* New York: NAL-Dutton, 1988.

Lappe, Frances M., ed. *Diet for a Small Planet.* New York: Ballantine Books, 1991.

Rombauer, Irma S. *Joy of Cooking.* New York: NAL-Dutton, 1991.

RENAL:

Gourmet Renal Nutrition Cookbook
Meredith Green, RD
Dialysis Unit
Lenox Hill Hospital
100 E. Seventy-seventh St.
New York, NY 10021

The Renal Family Cookbook
American Kidney Foundation
7315 Wisconsin Ave.
Bethesda, MD 20814

Kind Reader,

As the millennium approaches, your author is struggling to get with the program. By the time you read this, with luck, I will be on-line, e-mail address: http://www.critpath.org/cfl

Your patience is appreciated as any glitches get worked out.

Index